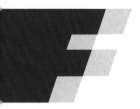

FAST FACTS

Indispensable

Guides to

Clinical

Practice

Cathy Speed

Consultant Rheumatologist and Director,
Sports and Exercise Medicine Unit,
Addenbrooke's Hospital, Cambridge, UK

Brian Hazleman

Consultant Rheumatologist and Director,
Rheumatology Research Unit,
Addenbrooke's Hospital, Cambridge, UK

Seamus Dalton

Consultant in Rehabilitation and
Sports Medicine, North Sydney Orthopaedic
& Sports Medicine Centre, Sydney, Australia

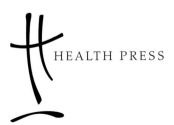

HEALTH PRESS

Oxford

Fast Facts – Soft Tissue Rheumatology
First published 2001

Text © 2001 Cathy Speed, Brian Hazleman, Seamus Dalton
© 2001 in this edition Health Press Limited
Elizabeth House, Queen Street, Abingdon, Oxford OX14 3JR, UK
Tel: +44 (0)1235 523233
Fax: +44 (0)1235 523238

Fast Facts is a trade mark of Health Press Limited.

The publisher and the authors have made every effort to ensure the
accuracy of this book, but cannot accept responsibility for any errors
or omissions.

A CIP catalogue record for this title is available from the British Library.

ISBN 1-899541-38-1

Speed, C (Cathy)
Fast Facts – Soft Tissue Rheumatology/
Cathy Speed, Brian Hazleman, Seamus Dalton

Illustrated by Dee McLean, London, UK.

Printed by Fine Print (Services) Ltd, Oxford, UK.

Introduction

Soft tissue injuries are common and of major importance as they are often a cause of significant morbidity and socioeconomic impact. In the UK alone, the resultant loss of working days from soft tissue lesions amounts to a cost of £1 billion every year in lost productivity, excluding the cost of related healthcare and social services, social security payments and lost tax revenue.

There is a general lack of understanding of many soft tissue complaints. This is probably related to the absence of a universally accepted system for classification of such disorders, their aetiologies, diagnosis and management. Perhaps as a result, the epidemiology of the majority of soft tissue disorders remains poorly defined. However, our understanding is improving steadily due to increased awareness, a growing acceptance of specific diagnostic criteria and advances in imaging techniques. Research by scientists with a specific interest in tendinopathies and soft tissue healing is also making a substantial contribution to advancing the approaches to classification and management of soft tissue disorders.

In this book, some of the issues surrounding soft tissue disorders are addressed. We begin by covering the structure of the major soft tissues and their common pathologies, and then explain the current classification system and discuss some commonly encountered conditions. Inevitably, not every soft tissue disorder has been included here, but the principles described in relation to those disorders discussed can be extrapolated to many other soft tissue complaints.

CHAPTER 1
Pathophysiology and epidemiology

Soft tissue rheumatology encompasses all musculoskeletal disorders that are not directly due to articular pathology. It includes disorders of:
- tendons and their sheaths
- ligaments
- bursae
- joint capsules
- muscles
- fascia.

Structure of soft tissue

Tendons and ligaments. The structures of tendons and ligaments are very similar; they are composed mainly of type I collagen fibrils, small amounts of type III collagen, elastin, fibrocytes, water and glycosaminoglycans. The latter form proteoglycans on binding to proteins.

A simplified description of the hierarchical structure of the tendon is shown in Figure 1.1. The fascicles, composed of groups of fibres, along with neurovascular structures and lymphatics, are surrounded by a loose connective tissue layer, the endotenon. Bundles of fascicles are surrounded by another connective tissue layer, the epitenon, and a double-layered covering, the paratenon. In some tendons, this covering may become a fluid-filled synovial sheath, the tenosynovium. Those tendons that have tenosynovial sheaths usually travel through narrow areas, such as the tendons of the hand and wrist, and those at the ankle (such as the peroneal tendons). Ligaments do not have sheaths.

Bursae are thin fluid-filled sacs that minimize friction between adjacent moving structures. They consist of fibrovascular tissue lined by synovium and are filled with a synovial-like fluid.

Joint capsules consist of fibrous collagenous tissue with some synovial lining.

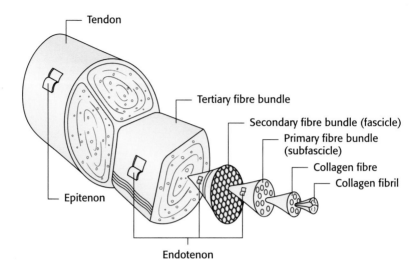

Figure 1.1 The hierarchical structure of tendon. The fascicles are composed of groups of fibres. The endotenon is a loose, connective tissue layer that surrounds the fascicles, neurovascular structures and lymphatics. The tertiary bundles of fascicles are surrounded by another connective tissue layer, the epitenon, and a double-layered covering, the paratenon (not shown).

Skeletal muscle. There are more than 430 voluntary muscles in the body. Skeletal muscle is made up of approximately 75% water, 20% protein and 5% salts, enzymes and other substances. Each muscle is composed of long cylindrical multinucleated cells (fibres) in parallel alignment. Each cell is surrounded by an elastic membrane (the sarcolemma) enclosing aqueous sarcoplasm within which the nuclei, contractile proteins, enzymes, glycogen, fat, other substances, and an intricate structural and transportation system of tubules (sarcoplasmic reticulum) are found (Figure 1.2).

Each fibre is wrapped in a fine layer of connective tissue (the endomysium). Bundles of fibres are wrapped together in another layer of connective tissue (the perimysium) to form fascicles. These are in turn bundled together within another layer (the epimysium) to form the muscle itself. Skeletal muscle has an extensive and complex blood supply that can be improved by physical training.

For detailed information on the gross structure and ultrastructure of skeletal muscle, readers are referred to the Key references section.

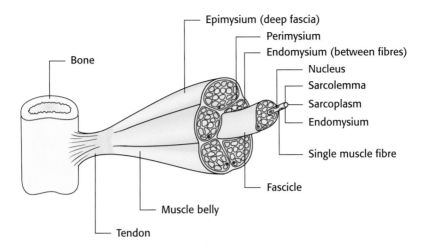

Figure 1.2 The structure of skeletal muscle.

Tendon mechanics

The mechanical behaviour of tendons is associated with the elasticity of the tissue and the *collagen crimp*. The latter refers to the wave-like shape of the collagen fascicles, which straightens on loading (Figure 1.3).

Pathophysiology

Soft tissue injuries can be described according to their duration at presentation, where:

- acute refers to a duration of less than 4 weeks
- subacute, 4–6 weeks
- chronic, lasting more than 6 weeks. Alternatively, a chronic injury can be defined as an acute injury occurring in association with some impairment to healing.

Most soft tissue tendon injuries are traumatic in origin.

- A macrotraumatic injury involves a single episode of acute tissue destruction.
- A microtraumatic injury involves either chronic overload or an acute-on-chronic episode. This may be due to intrinsic and/or extrinsic factors causing inflammation, degeneration, tear or rupture.

9

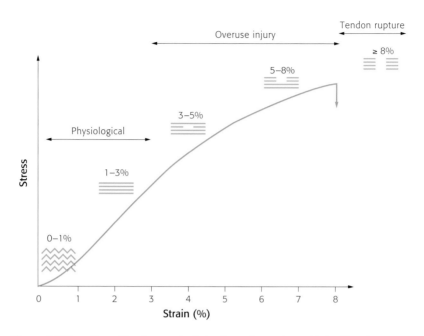

Figure 1.3 The effect of loading on the behaviour of a tendon. With loading, the collagen fibrils realign and undergo elastic deformation, returning to their original structure and length when unloaded if the forces are not too severe. If the load is too great, injury occurs and the original structure will not be regained (plastic deformation). As the load is increased, rupture occurs. The force level at which this occurs is related to the cross-sectional area and length of the tendon.

Ligament injuries. Ligament sprains can be graded from I (mild, with no instability) to III (complete tear with instability).

Tendon injuries. Rupture of a healthy tendon is relatively rare, but occurs in tendons that are already abnormal – for example, those that have been injured previously or where there is degeneration within the central tendon substance (which may be subclinical up to the point of rupture). Degenerate tendon rupture can occur asymptomatically and is often attritional, for example at the long head of biceps or the Achilles tendon. Certain conditions and drugs are associated with tendon injury (Table 1.1).

Knowledge of the pathological features of a tendon injury allows combined clinical and histological grading of tendinopathies (Table 1.2).

TABLE 1.1

Systemic disorders and drugs associated with tendon disorders

- Inflammatory and crystal arthropathies
- Diabetes mellitus
- Oestrogen deficiency (including menopause)
- Drugs: glucocorticoids, fluoroquinolone antibiotics, anabolic steroids
- Any joint pathology that may alter biomechanics
- ? Stress and overtraining: increased circulating glucocorticoids and catecholamines

Response to acute injury

Tissue response to acute injury involves specific processes. Various outcomes are possible, depending upon both intrinsic and extrinsic factors. These processes are listed in Table 1.3.

Inflammation is a time-dependent, localized and *necessary* tissue response to injury (Table 1.4). It involves vascular, chemical and cellular events, leading to tissue repair, regeneration or scar formation. Excessive inflammation is deleterious. Although pain is often assumed to represent inflammation, this is not always the case as the origin of connective tissue pain is multifactorial (Figure 1.4).

Healing. There are three potential outcomes – resolution, repair and remodelling/maturation.

Resolution involves the reversal of vascular changes and the removal of fibrin, exudate and dead cells, so that the original tissue structure is regained. This is the optimal outcome, but it rarely occurs.

Repair of soft tissue injury usually involves the replacement of damaged/lost cells and extracellular matrices. It can involve *regeneration* or, more commonly, *organization*. Regeneration is a form of repair that produces new tissue structurally and functionally identical to normal tissue. Tissues differ in their ability to regenerate. The regenerative capacity of bone and fibrous tissues is good, while that of skeletal

11

TABLE 1.2

Classification of tendon disorders*

Disorder	Definition
Paratenonitis**	Inflammation of paratenon ± synovium
Paratenonitis and tendinosis	Inflammation of paratenon and intratendinous degeneration
Tendinosis	Intratendinous degeneration
Tendinitis	Symptomatic degeneration with vascular disruption and inflammatory response
Tear	Disruption of tendon integrity

*Adapted from Clancy 1990 and Puddu *et al.* 1976
**Tenosynovitis is included in this term, as is tenovaginitis, which expresses an additional restriction of the tendon due to scarring or adhesions within the sheath

muscle and nerve tissue is poor. Organization involves the formation of scar tissue via granulation and subsequent fibrosis. The histological and biomechanical properties of scar tissue differ from those of the original tissue.

Remodelling/maturation of new tissue occurs over weeks or months, in response to loading and biomechanical stresses.

Histology	Clinical
• Inflammation-associated cells in paratenon/peritendinous tissue	• Swelling • Pain • Crepitus • Local warmth • Dysfunction
As above **plus** • Fibre disarray • Decreased cellularity • Vascular ingrowth • Calcification	• As above • ± Nodule
• Fibre disarray • Decreased cellularity • Vascular ingrowth • Calcification	• ± Nodule • ± Point tenderness
• Acute inflammation • Inflammation on degeneration • Calcification and degeneration • ± Central necrosis • ± Interstitial injury	• Signs of inflammation • ± Nodule • ± Point tenderness
As tendinosis/tendinitis	• Pain • Poor response to treatment • Weakness • Palpable gap

If the injury is a total rupture or a significant tear, the constant tension on the tendon from the attached muscle may prevent satisfactory healing; the gap between the ends must be closed, and surgery may be required. A tendon also needs to maintain a gliding function; so healing within the tissue without adherence to other tissues is important. Early mobilization is vital, but excess joint motion or excessive forces through the tendon may be deleterious.

TABLE 1.3

Tissue responses to acute injury

- Inflammation
- Healing
  - resolution
  - repair
    - regeneration
    - organization, e.g. granulation, fibrosis
- Remodelling/maturation

TABLE 1.4

Cardinal signs of inflammation

Sign	Process
Heat (calor)	• Metabolic energy
Redness (rubor)	• Increased blood flow
Swelling (tumor)	• Extracellular oedema and matrix changes
Pain (dolor)	• Noxious mediators causing stimulation of afferent nerve endings
Loss of function (functio laesa) which may manifest as weakness, stiffness or decreased performance	• Any combination of the above

Factors affecting response to injury

In the successful management of acute soft tissue injury, the responses that promote efficient optimal recovery should be maximized, and the adverse responses limited. Factors that influence response are shown in Table 1.5. Most of those factors that predispose to injury have the potential to impair the response to the event(s).

Chronic inflammation is usually related to microtraumatic injury. In a highly innervated, vascular connective tissue environment, leucocytes become

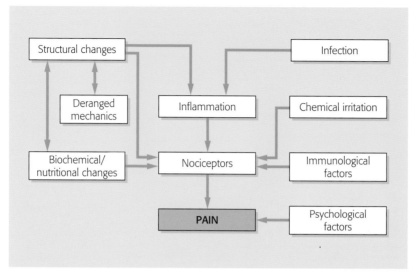

Figure 1.4 Sources of musculoskeletal pain.

TABLE 1.5

Factors affecting response to tissue injury

- Apposition of torn tissue ends
- Inflammation is part of the healing process but excessive inflammation is deleterious
- Activity – early controlled activity is helpful, but excessive activity may impair recovery
- Age – tissues take longer to heal with increasing age, partly as a result of morphological and biochemical changes in collagen and elastin fibres
- Nutrition – adequate protein, energy, vitamins and minerals are important
- Vascularity – a poor vascular supply may be important in the chronicity of soft tissue injuries such as tendon disorders
- Endocrine factors – hypoestrogenism may be associated with an increased incidence of tendinosis, while the poor healing response in diabetes is well recognized
- Genetic factors may influence the predisposition to injuries and the nature and speed of the response
- Innervation

replaced by macrophages, plasma cells and lymphocytes. A common factor contributing to inflammation is the continued overloading of acutely damaged tissue, resulting in changes in local cellular activity.

Degeneration is a change in tissue to a less functionally active form, which is then more prone to injury. This phenomenon can result from immobilization, increased age, denervation, poor nutrition and persistent inflammation.

Epidemiology

Local soft tissue disorders constitute a significant demand on both primary care and hospital services. The lack of universally acceptable diagnostic criteria for many soft tissue disorders has been the major factor in the lack of epidemiological studies of such complaints. Although the precise incidence and prevalence of such disorders are difficult to define, soft tissue lesions are considered to represent one-third of all rheumatic diseases seen

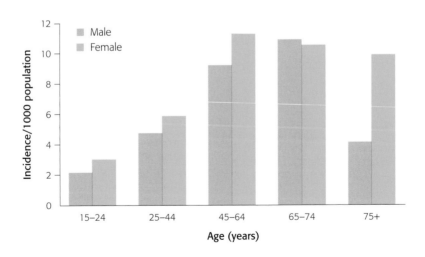

Figure 1.5 Estimated incidence of shoulder symptoms (all causes) in the UK. Reproduced from the Royal College of Practitioners. Office of Population Censuses and Surveys. Department of Health and Social Security. Morbidity statistics from general practice. Second National Study 1971–1972, London: HMSO, 1979 and Third National Study 1981–1982, London: HMSO, 1986.

by family physicians. They are the most common rheumatic causes of sickness absences from work, accounting for 44% of certified rheumatic episodes and 6% of the total number of episodes of incapacity. This represents 3.5% of all days lost from work and, in the UK alone, almost £1 billion in lost productivity annually, excluding the cost of social security payments, lost tax reserve and cost to health and social services.

The prevalence of all forms of soft tissue rheumatism is difficult to assess but has been estimated at 1.6% in men and 3.6% in women. Of all localized problems, the painful shoulder ranks highest in frequency. In the UK, at least 1 in 170 of the adult population will present to their family physician with a new episode of shoulder pain each year; most episodes are due to soft tissue lesions. The estimated incidence of all shoulder symptoms in the UK is shown in Figure 1.5.

CHAPTER 2
Classification and diagnosis

As pain is the primary symptom of soft tissue disorders, its site and distribution are suitable criteria for classification. Soft tissue disorders can be described as either diffuse (generalized or regional) or local (according to the specific site). The tissue that is affected, pathology involved and aetiology (Table 2.1) are all important (Figure 2.1). Examples of how soft tissue disorders might usefully be described are shown in Table 2.2. Additional information from clinical findings, imaging studies and laboratory investigations is also useful.

General features of soft tissue injuries

Pain. The cardinal symptom of a soft tissue disorder is pain that can arise from many sources (see Figure 1.4, page 15).

TABLE 2.1

Aetiology of soft tissue injuries

Intrinsic

- Biomechanical: anatomical and/or functional malalignments
- Muscle imbalance
- Poor technique
- Hypermobility
- Hypomobility
- Poor vascular supply
- Disease
- Fatigued muscles (altered movement patterns)

Others

- Immobilization (tissue atrophy, weakness)
- Local steroid injection (mechanical disruption, reduced collagen synthesis)
- ?Non-steroidal anti-inflammatory drugs (can mask injury)

Extrinsic

- Equipment, e.g. poor heel counter causes Achilles tendinitis
- Training patterns (sudden increase in intensity/volume)
- Surface
- Environment, e.g. extremes of temperature

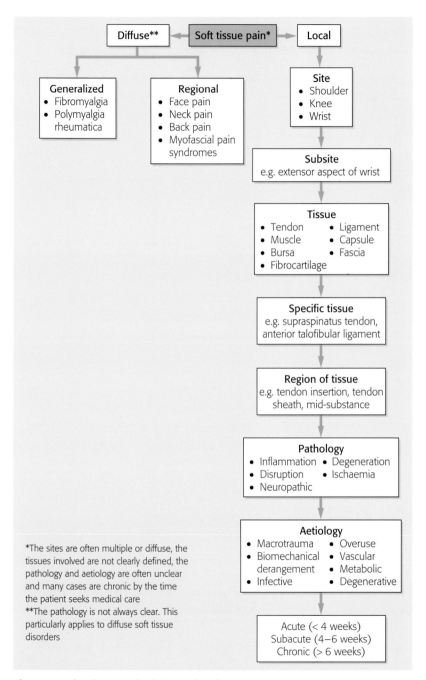

Figure 2.1 Classification of soft tissue disorders.

TABLE 2.2

Examples of useful clinical descriptions of soft tissue disorders

Partial tear of the rotator cuff secondary to rotator cuff tendinitis secondary to impingement secondary to instability of the glenohumeral joint

A local soft tissue disorder

- Site: shoulder

- Tissue: tendon, rotator cuff

- Pathology: disruption, inflammation (?), attempts to repair, degeneration

- Aetiology: impingement, instability

Lateral ankle sprain

A local soft tissue disorder

- Site: lateral ankle

- Tissue: ligaments; anterior talofibular ± calcaneofibular ± posterior talofibular

- Pathology: disruption, graded I to III, and inflammation

- Aetiology: trauma and, for example, imbalance due to weak peroneal muscles

Localized soft tissue injuries, particularly those affecting tendons, often have a characteristic pain cycle (Figure 2.2). In low-grade injury, soft tissue pain initially disappears during the first few minutes of use and activity proceeds. Pain returns after activity but is usually not severe enough to prevent activity the next day. Eventually, the pain does not disappear during activity and limits function. Only relative rest and appropriate intervention to treat the injury will help to break the pain cycle.

A grading system for pain, based on pain arising from tendon injuries, is shown in Table 2.3.

Symptoms of inflammation may be present in acute, chronic or acute-on-chronic injuries, but are not universally present.

Clicking may be related to instability, inflammation, a tear or to scarring after an injury, but in the absence of other symptoms may be clinically irrelevant.

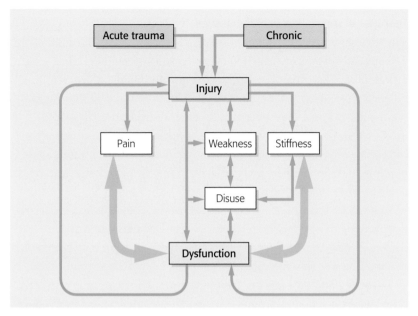

Figure 2.2 Pain cycle in soft tissue injury.

Stiffness is also a common feature of soft tissue injuries and may be related to local swelling, fibrosis and scarring. It returns after exercise in chronic injuries.

Dysfunction is a frequent and important result of soft tissue injury and may be related to instability, gross disruption of the tissue, more subtle biomechanical alterations or to pain itself (see Figure 1.4, page 15).

TABLE 2.3

Grades of pain in local soft tissue disorders

Grade	Characteristics
I	Pain only occurs on extreme exertion and ceases when activity stops
II	Pain occurs with moderate activity, but disappears after a short time; it reappears after cessation of activity and persists for 1–2 hours
III	Pain is present with any activity and may persist for many hours afterwards
IV	Pain present at rest

Features of injuries to specific tissues

Tendon injuries can be classified according to the guidelines in Figure 2.1. The presenting features of a tendon disorder will depend on the timing of presentation. There may be some overlap in clinical findings between different types of tendon injury, particularly in chronic conditions. Acute injuries may present with some or all of the classical features described above. Unfortunately, a unifying feature of chronic tendon disorders is their complexity of symptoms and signs. Imaging studies are often helpful, but histological information is rarely available. Some of the common features of tendinopathies are shown in Table 2.4.

Some of the features of an acute inflammatory tendinopathy, particularly dysfunction, may be present in chronic injuries. However, pain and tenderness may be poorly localized and inflammatory signs may be absent, as not all chronic soft tissue injuries involve chronic inflammation.

Triggering may be a feature. Triggering is a feeling of locking, often of a digit, usually due to local tendon scarring. The joint will unlock with effort or on passively moving the joint. The patient may complain of clicking or snapping when unlocking occurs.

Nodules. A solid nodule may be palpable and may be associated with triggering. A bulbous swelling may be evident close to a point of constriction.

Tendon rupture is usually associated with an acute episode of pain and dysfunction during activity. The precipitating activity may be relatively minor if the tendon is degenerate and/or has been injured in the past. The patient often reports an audible snap, followed by pain, haemorrhage and inflammation in the area surrounding the ruptured area and dysfunction. Weakness out of proportion to pain and a palpable gap may be evident. Tendon rupture can occur asymptomatically in a degenerate tendon (e.g. the long head of the biceps).

Enthesopathies. An enthesopathy is a disorder of the enthesis, the site where the tendon or ligament inserts into bone. Ossification at this site may be a feature. Symptoms depend upon the site involved. Enthesopathies can be classified according to whether they are inflammatory, traumatic, metabolic or degenerative in origin (or a combination of more than one of these types). Enthesopathies are known to be a feature of spondyloarthritides (Table 2.5).

TABLE 2.4

Common features of tendinopathies

Symptoms	Signs

• Local pain
  – may vary from a constant ache to sharp stabbing pain with movement
  – radiates proximally or distally from lesion
  – worsens with use, work against resistance and passive stretching
  – occurs while resting in severe cases
	• Local pain
	  – local tenderness
	  – worsens with testing against resistance and with passive stretching

• Swelling	• Swelling
	  – diffuse or localized
	  – palpable nodule may be present

• Dysfunction	• Dysfunction – weakness is often in proportion to pain but when it is out of proportion to pain consider that a tear in the tendon may be present

• Other symptoms of inflammation	• Other signs of inflammation
	  – redness
	  – warmth

• 'Creaking'	• Crepitus
• Appropriate precipitating event(s)	• Predisposing features, e.g. biomechanical malalignment

Ligament injuries. In addition to the guidelines in Figure 2.1, ligament injuries ('sprains') can be further defined as grades I–III (Table 2.6). Pain, bruising and swelling are common in acute injuries, while clicking and subjective or true mechanical instability are more common in chronic injuries.

Other injuries may occur in association with ligament damage and must always be considered when assessing the patient. For example in ankle sprains, avulsion injuries and syndesmosis tears can occur.

TABLE 2.5

Spondyloarthritides associated with enthesopathies

- Ankylosing spondylitis
- Psoriatic arthritis
- Reiter's syndrome/reactive arthropathy
- Seronegative enthesopathic arthropathy syndrome
- Undifferentiated spondylitis
- Enteropathic arthritis (Crohn's disease, ulcerative colitis)

TABLE 2.6

Ligament injuries*

Grade	Description	Clinical findings**
I	Microscopic damage to ligament	• Localized pain and tenderness • Pain on stressing ligament • No joint instability
II	Partial tear of ligament	• Localized pain and tenderness • Pain on stressing ligament • Mild joint instability with firm end-point • Joint swelling if tear is intracapsular
III	Complete tear of ligament Ligament or bony avulsion	• Localized pain and tenderness • Bruising and swelling • Unstable joint • No end-point • Pain often absent on stressing the ligament

*These can occur mid-substance or at the bony insertions
**Inflammation may also be present

Disorders of bursae. Bursae are thin, fluid-filled sacs that minimize friction between adjacent moving structures. They can be situated between tendons, between tendon and bone, or beneath skin at bony prominences. There are over 80 natural bursae on each side of the body. Palpable bursae are an indication that pathology is (or has been) present. Pathological bursae can develop as a result of trauma or excessive friction, direct or systemic sepsis, or in association with inflammatory and crystal arthropathies. When inflammation is present, the term 'bursitis' is applied (Table 2.7). Pathological bursae may be further described according to their site (superficial or deep) and aetiology. At least 12 bursae are found in the region of the knee and are described in Figure 2.3.

Clinical features. There may be a history of acute trauma or repetitive overuse. The possibility of sepsis and systemic disease must always be considered. Often the presence of bursitis indicates the existence of a more complex problem. For example, rotator cuff disorders can be associated with subacromial bursitis, while trochanteric bursitis can be associated with pelvic instability and muscle weakness.

Superficial, pathological bursae may be visible as localized, well-defined swellings, often with associated inflammation, pain on local palpation and crepitus.

Deeper, pathological bursae are more difficult to diagnose clinically. Pain may occur on passive stretching of the surrounding tissues and/or on local compression of the area. Imaging may be necessary to confirm the diagnosis.

Infective bursitis should be considered if there is a history of systemic upset, fever, direct inoculation into the bursa through trauma, or in any patient who has a systemic disease and/or is immunosuppressed. *Staphylococcus aureus* or other Gram-positive cocci are most commonly involved, although Gram-negative organisms are often seen in patients with

TABLE 2.7

Causes of bursitis

- Trauma (acute or chronic)
- Sepsis
- Metabolic/crystals
- Calcific deposits
- Inflammatory arthritides
- Idiopathic

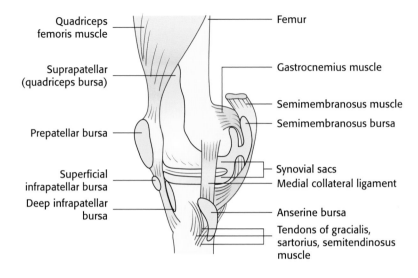

Figure 2.3 Distribution of bursae around the knee (medial view). These include the suprapatellar, prepatellar, infrapatellar and adventitious cutaneous bursae anteriorly; the gastrocnemius and semimembranosus bursae posteriorly; three bursae adjacent to the fibular collateral ligament and the popliteal tendon laterally; and the sartorius and anserine bursae and a bursa near to the medial collateral ligament medially (not all shown).

systemic disorders. The major differential diagnosis in this situation is a crystal-induced bursitis.

Imaging

The presence of many soft tissue disorders can usually be determined clinically. However, imaging may be required when a significant tear or focal tendon lesion is suspected, or to define contributing anatomical structures. The full nature and extent of the injury and additional underlying pathologies can be determined by imaging studies. Sensitive imaging techniques also allow more accurate classification of tendon disorders.

Magnetic resonance imaging (MRI) and ultrasound are the gold standards for investigating local soft tissue disorders. They have the advantages of providing multiplanar images in real time without exposure to radiation. MRI has the advantage over ultrasound of allowing imaging of any anatomical structure or location (Figure 2.4). It provides excellent multiplanar imaging of anatomical structures and T1- and T2-weighted images, and fat-suppressed and proton-dense views provide information about bone oedema, blood or water content and muscle atrophy. The disadvantages of MRI are that it is more expensive and less commonly available than other forms of imaging.

Ultrasonography is quick, inexpensive and provides real-time dynamic imaging. It also allows easy comparison with the asymptomatic limb or joint. It is more commonly available than MRI, but its value is extremely user-dependent, particularly in the case of shoulder ultrasound. With improving technology, ultrasound is becoming increasingly sensitive.

Ultrasonography is also being used as an alternative to fluoroscopy for accurate aspiration or injection of cysts, haematomas, ganglia and areas of calcific tendinitis (Figure 2.5). It allows accurate intra-articular injection where blind access can be difficult (e.g. in the hip and glenohumeral joints), and it negates the need for radiographic dye.

Computerized tomography (CT) may be used, often in conjunction with arthrography, but involves radiation and has few advantages over MRI other than possibly cost and availability.

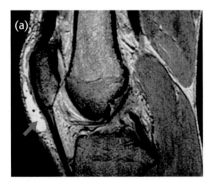 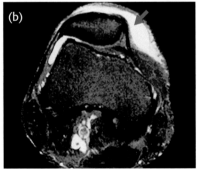

Figure 2.4 (a) A T2-weighted MR image showing a large prepatellar bursa (arrowed) in a marathon runner. Note the high-signal intensity due to the fluid content. (b) Fluid (arrowed) was also seen within the joint.

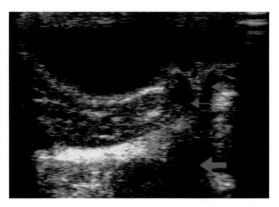

Figure 2.5 An ultrasound scan of a semimembranosus gastrocnemius bursa (popliteal or Baker's cyst) (large arrow). Note the anechoic structure representing the cyst arising and pouting between the medial head of the gastrocnemius and the tendon for semi-membranosus laterally (thin arrows). This is characteristic of a Baker's cyst and confirms the diagnosis.

Radiographs. Plain radiographs need not be performed routinely but allow confirmation or can help to exclude bony pathology, for example in the exclusion of an underlying fracture in an ankle sprain (see Table 4.2, page 44). Radiographs also allow identification of any anatomical features that may be contributing to the injury or condition (e.g. an acromial spur in rotator cuff tendinitis contributing to subacromial impingement, or a Haglund's deformity in retrocalcaneal bursitis and Achilles tendinitis). In skilled hands, soft tissue radiographs reveal not only areas of calcification but also thickening of tissues such as the patellar and Achilles tendons.

Arthrography may be used to confirm the presence of a rotator cuff tear (Figure 2.6), or ligament disruption in wrist injuries, and can aid in the diagnosis of adhesive capsulitis.

CT arthrography is useful in the identification of labral and capsular pathologies in the shoulder. Wear of the glenoid, fractures and loose bodies are also best imaged using CT.

Radionucleotide imaging (bone scans) can be useful in the investigation of enthesopathies or to exclude osseous or joint pathology. For local or

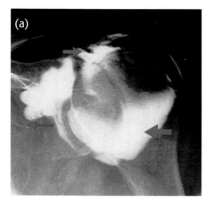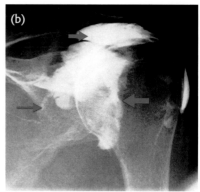

Figure 2.6 (a) An arthrogram of the left shoulder showing a very tight joint (large arrow) and filling of the lymphatics (thin arrow). (b) Note that contrast has escaped into the subacromial/subdeltoid bursa (small arrow), which confirms the connection between the bursa and the joint, indicating a full-thickness tear through the rotator cuff tendons, usually the supraspinatus tendon.

regional pain disorders, in which the underlying pathology is not apparent but bone pain is suspected, isotope scanning may be needed to exclude sinister pathology such as neoplastic disease.

CHAPTER 3
Management guidelines

Successful management of soft tissue disorders requires:
- early recognition
- identification of the cause(s)
- treatment of specific pathology/pathologies.

In all soft tissue injuries, the following should be considered:
- what was the mechanism of injury?
- when did it occur (i.e. is it an acute or chronic injury)?
- what are the underlying potentiating factors?

Tendon injuries

Although various parts of the tendon structure may be damaged in a tendon injury, most tendon disorders are managed along the same basic guidelines (Table 3.1). Exceptions to this are the ruptured tendon and the significant tear, which may require a prompt surgical opinion.

In chronic injuries, it may be difficult to define the stage of repair that the tissue has reached. If in doubt, treat as an acute injury, starting with the 'PRICES-MM' approach.

TABLE 3.1

Management approach for tendon injuries*

Stage of healing	Time (days)	Suggested therapy
Inflammatory	0–6	PRICES-MM
Fibroblastic/proliferative	5–21	Gradual introduction of stress
Remodelling/maturation	20+	Progressive stress on tissue at a rate determined by the individual's response without exacerbating symptoms

*Adapted from el Hawary et al. 1997

PRICES-MM approach. Excessive inflammation can be limited by adopting this approach in the first 24–48 hours after injury:

- Protect
- Rest the injured area
- Ice (10–20 minutes every 2–4 hours)
- Compress
- Elevate
- Support
- Modalities. The most frequently used modality in tendon injuries is *ice*, which has anti-inflammatory and analgesic actions. *Ultrasound* is often used in soft tissue injuries, although currently there is no good evidence to support its use. When ultrasound waves are applied to soft tissue, they produce absorbable energy with 'thermal' and/or 'non-thermal' effects. Thermal effects include increasing soft tissue extensibility, decreasing tissue stiffness and muscle spasm, increased blood flow and modulation of pain. Excessive heating of the tissue with high-intensity ultrasound may cause local tissue damage. Experimental evidence suggests that ultrasound may speed resolution of inflammation, accelerate fibroblast function, accelerate angiogenesis and increase matrix synthesis and the strength of healing tissues – such effects are considered 'non-thermal'. If the ultrasound intensity is low, only non-thermal effects occur.

Physiological rationale	Main goals
• Prevent excessive inflammation • Prevent disruption of new blood vessels and collagen fibrils • Promote synthesis of ground substance	• Promote healing • Avoid new tissue disruption
• Promote normal biomechanical integrity of tendon structure	• Prevent excessive tissue atrophy
• Promote normal biomechanical integrity of tendon structure	• Optimize tissue healing

Ultrasound can be delivered in the form of continuous or pulsed (on–off) waves. Continuous waves have a greater thermal effect, whilst pulsed waves are used more frequently since they incur less tissue damage. *Laser* therapy has similar effects to ultrasound but decreases inflammation and may be useful in superficial injuries

- Medication if necessary – simple analgesics and non-steroidal anti-inflammatory drugs (NSAIDs), see below.

Note that inflammation is a homeostatic mechanism and is part of the body's natural response to injury. However, excessive or prolonged inflammation can be damaging, limiting vascular supply and impairing rehabilitation due to pain and restriction. Dampening the inflammatory process may assist healing when inflammation is excessive, but may inhibit healing if inflammation is moderate.

Other management techniques

Acupuncture and transcutaneous electrical nerve stimulation (TENS) may also be helpful in the management of pain, particularly that resulting from chronic soft tissue injuries.

Resting splints, used intermittently, are often very useful for the prevention of soft tissue shortening while healing is taking place. They can also stop excessive movement.

Pharmacotherapy

NSAIDs are among the most commonly prescribed drugs and are often overused. They should be used only when inflammation is present and is considered to be impairing the healing process. Proposed mechanisms of action include:

- inhibition of cyclo-oxygenase (COX)
- inhibition of the release of numerous inflammatory mediators and destructive agents
- interference with interaction between inflammatory cells
- promotion of fibrinolysis
- reduction of platelet aggregation and platelet-derived growth factor.

Side-effects associated with NSAIDs are common and varied (Table 3.2). Most seriously, gastrointestinal and renal toxicity may occur, particularly among elderly users.

Which NSAID? It is not possible to be dogmatic about individual NSAIDs. Differences between NSAIDs lie mainly in the incidence and type of side-effects, as variation in anti-inflammatory effect is frequently small. Interindividual variation in response is significant, however, and trials of several different NSAIDs may be necessary. The selective COX-2 inhibitors, such as rofecoxib and celecoxib, may be associated with a reduced incidence of side-effects.

Using topical preparations (some are available over the counter) can also significantly reduce the risk of side-effects; these are particularly useful in superficial lesions. Patients should be warned that systemic side-effects, such as gastrointestinal disturbance, and local skin sensitivity can occur, and be advised to apply small amounts of the gel to the injured area four or five

TABLE 3.2

Side-effects of non-steroidal anti-inflammatory drugs

Gastrointestinal

- Dyspepsia
- Ulceration
- Haemorrhage
- Perforation

Renal

- Acute renal failure (reversible or irreversible)
- Increased blood pressure
- Cardiac failure

Hepatic

- Variable, e.g. 'transaminitis'

Hypersensitivity

- Rashes
- Bronchospasm

Haematological

- Haemolysis
- Thrombocytopenia
- Neutropenia
- Red cell aplasia

Drug interactions

- Reduced efficacy, e.g. diuretics, antihypertensive agents
- Increased efficacy, e.g. anticonvulsants, digoxin, anticoagulants, lithium

times daily, massaging the gel thoroughly into the area. The effect of local massage with the gel may also be of benefit.

Steroid injections. Local corticosteroids have no role in the management of acute injuries, and are not indicated in most ligament lesions. They are useful in the management of chronic soft tissue injuries, particularly tendinopathies and bursitis, but must be used judiciously and are not the first-line approach to treatment. Steroid injections should be used when other recommended approaches have been unsuccessful. Guidelines for the use of local steroids in tendon injury are given in Table 3.3. Guidelines for some specific disorders are given in Table 3.4.

Potential side-effects include:
- tissue atrophy
- inflammatory flare
- hypersensitivity
- serious complications, including sepsis.

Some local corticosteroids may cause alterations of the structural characteristics of ligament and tendon when injected into their substance. These can include weakening of the structure and decreased stiffness, reduced energy absorption and load to failure. The effects of local corticosteroids may be related to the:
- type of steroid used
- tissue involved
- extent of the injury
- stage of healing at time of injection
- post-injection events, particularly loading of the tissue.

Injudicious loading of soft tissue structures soon after local steroid injections increases the risk of significant injury. Complete tendon rupture with loading has often been reported in individuals who have had a prior steroid injection.

Local anaesthetic injections, without corticosteroid, are often useful for diagnostic purposes. It is possible that, in some lesions, dry injection is as effective as injecting local steroids and/or anaesthetic (see Regional myofascial pain syndromes, pages 86–7).

TABLE 3.3

Guidelines for the use of local steroids in tendon injury

Indications (all should be present)

- Chronic injury in which conservative management has failed and sites where inflammatory processes are evident **plus**

- Inhibited rehabilitation (having detrimental effects on soft tissue structures) **plus**

- The patient should be willing to comply with post-injection guidelines

Practical measures

- Exclude infection prior to injection

- Use aseptic technique

- Use short-acting preparations in most cases

- Use with local anaesthetic

- Avoid injecting into tendon substance

- A minimum of 2 weeks' post-injection rest is necessary

- An interval of at least 6 weeks is required between injections

- The maximum number of injections for any patient is three

Other considerations

- In heavily loaded tendons, consider an MRI or ultrasound scan to exclude deeper (central) injury or focal degeneration prior to injection

- The authors do not recommend local steroid injections in the vicinity of the Achilles or patellar tendons

- Soluble preparations may be useful in those patients who have had a hypersensitivity local reaction to a previous injection

- Local corticosteroids are often unnecessary in the younger patient

- If pain relief and anti-inflammatory effects can be achieved by other methods, injections should be avoided

Above all

- Know the anatomy

- Know the injury

- Know your patient

- Advise your patient of possible complications

TABLE 3.4

Guidelines for local steroid injections for specific soft tissue disorders*

Disorder	Corticosteroid
Subacromial bursitis	Methylprednisolone acetate, 40 mg
Rotator cuff tendinitis (particularly with impingement)	Methylprednisolone acetate, 40 mg
Bicipital tendinitis	Hydrocortisone, ≤ 20 mg
Frozen shoulder	Methylprednisolone acetate, 40 mg
Medial/lateral epicondylitis	Hydrocortisone, ≤ 20 mg
Tenosynovitis of the wrist	Hydrocortisone, ≤ 20 mg
Trochanteric bursitis	Hydrocortisone, ≤ 20 mg
Plantar fasciitis	Hydrocortisone, ≤ 20 mg

*Readers are strongly advised to refer to specific texts and to obtain practical skills (with supervision by an experienced physician) on local injection techniques prior to performing these approaches
**A blue needle is appropriate in most cases

Exercise

Graded exercise is a fundamental part of the treatment programme for soft tissue injuries. Exercise can be started early, within 48 hours, in order to achieve a functional recovery and prevent further injury. The acronym REST – *R*esume *E*xercise below *S*oreness *T*hreshold – is a good guide to the intensity with which the patient should exercise.

Passive motion within a pain-free range is safe in the very early stages following injury, and will have beneficial effects on the injured tissues. After a warm-up, gentle static stretching should then be introduced, gradually working towards active exercise. An appropriate tensile loading programme should be started early to promote collagen synthesis, alignment, maturation and functional integrity. Loading can be gradually increased over time by increasing the number of repetitions and/or force involved. Selective prescription of eccentric and concentric exercises is needed to optimize recovery and restoration of function. The goal should be to work towards full, specific, pain-free functional activity. If pain occurs after the session, or the injury becomes exacerbated, reduce

Route**

Subacromial space (lateral approach)

Subacromial space (lateral approach)

Bicipital groove

Shoulder joint, anterior or posterior route

To point of maximum tenderness, near to bone

Into tendon sheath

With affected side uppermost, direct needle perpendicular to skin, towards site of maximum tenderness, near to trochanter. A longer needle may be necessary

Medial approach, to point of maximum tenderness, near to bone

the loading. All activity should be followed by further flexibility exercises. After cool-down exercises, ice should be applied to the injured area (Figure 3.1).

Proprioceptive training is paramount in conditions such as ankle sprains. Any muscle imbalances, which are particularly common among younger patients, must be assessed and considered when designing an exercise programme.

Lack of response

There may be several reasons for poor response to therapy. These include:

- incorrect diagnosis
- presence of a tear within the tendon substance
- poor compliance
- excessive loading during the exercise programme
- ongoing presence of exacerbating factors, such as incorrect equipment or biomechanical abnormalities.

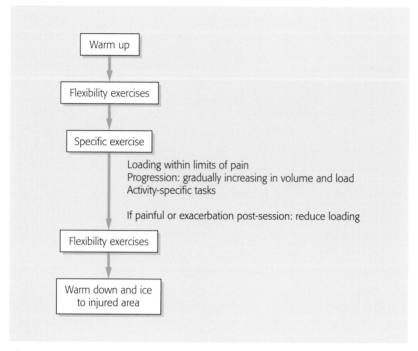

Figure 3.1 Graded exercise in soft tissue injuries.

Surgery

Surgery is usually avoidable for soft tissue disorders, but can be considered under some circumstances (Table 3.5).

Bursitis

Most uncomplicated episodes of bursitis will settle with relative rest, removal of the causative factor(s), protection (such as elbow pads) and NSAIDs, if necessary. Occasionally, aspiration of the bursa may be required and in itself may provide symptomatic relief. Intrabursal injection of corticosteroid may settle inflammation, but should be used only in resistant cases and when the clinician is confident that infection is not present. They may be useful in:
- resistant, chronic bursitis
- chronic, deep, frictional bursitis
- crystal-related bursitis, e.g. gout.

Surgical intervention for bursitis is rarely necessary.

TABLE 3.5

Occasions when surgery can be considered for soft tissue disorders

Investigation

- Arthroscopic surgery to investigate soft tissue disorders related to joint pathology

Repair of structures

- To repair total rupture of a structure, such as the Achilles tendon
- To repair tears within the tendon substance that have failed to heal and continue to prevent a positive response to conservative management

Excision of degenerate lesions or partial tears

- To resect mucoid degeneration in patellar tendinitis or chronic epicondylitis

Release of structures

- To release tight or scarred structures, e.g. lateral release for lateral epicondylitis when conservative management has failed
- To release an area of constriction surrounding a tendon
- To release persistent tendon triggering that occurs despite conservative management

Alteration of contributing anatomical structures

- On failure of conservative management in a tendinopathy where there is a precipitating mechanical cause, such as Haglund's deformity in retrocalcaneal bursitis

Instability

- Continuing mechanical and functional instability of a joint due to mechanical disruption of tissue(s), e.g. in some patients with cruciate ligament rupture
- With subluxation of tendons, e.g. peroneus longus, where the retinaculum is torn

Infective bursitis. Management includes aspiration to dryness of the bursa for urgent Gram stain and culture of the synovial fluid. Daily aspiration or surgical drainage will be required. *S. aureus* or other Gram-positive cocci are most commonly involved, although Gram-negative organisms are often seen in patients with systemic disorders. Where Gram-positive cocci have been identified, treatment should be started for penicillin-resistant *S. aureus* (with flucloxacillin 250–500 mg four times daily, for example) while awaiting culture results. If the patient is in good general health with little systemic upset and in the absence of overlying cellulitis, treatment may be in the form of oral antibiotics. All other patients should be treated with parenteral therapy, changing to oral therapy when an adequate response is evident. Treatment should be continued for 10–14 days, longer in immunosuppressed patients if necessary.

CHAPTER 4
Ankle sprains

Ankle sprains are one of the most common soft tissue injuries and their significance should never be underestimated. They are an important cause of long-term pain and dysfunction. Lateral ligament sprains as a result of an inversion injury are much more common than injuries to the medial ligament complex, which is one of the strongest ligaments in the body (Figure 4.1). Medial ligament injuries usually only occur with severe trauma.

Lateral ligament injuries
Defining the mechanism of injury is of paramount importance and provides an insight into the type and extent of the injury. The history is usually that of an inversion injury of the supinated, plantar-flexed foot. This is the position of least bony stability of the ankle, with the soft tissue structures supplying the support. The injury usually affects the anterior talofibular ligament, and may progress posteriorly to affect the calcaneofibular ligament, then the posterior talofibular ligament. The force applied as a result of body weight, momentum and foot position will influence the extent of the injury. Associated injuries must always be considered (Table 4.1).

(a)   (b)

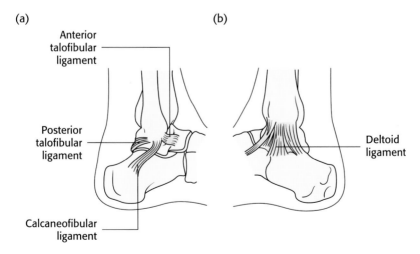

Figure 4.1 The ligaments of the ankle: (a) lateral view; (b) medial view.

TABLE 4.1

Additional injuries and complications in ankle sprains

- Fracture
- Osteochondral lesions to the talus or tibial plafond
- Peroneal tendon injuries (subluxation, tear, avulsion of peroneus brevis)
- Peroneal muscle weakness
- Tibialis posterior tendon injury
- Disruption of the distal tibiofibular syndesmosis
- Chronic synovitis
- Nerve traction injury (particularly peroneal nerve)
- Reflex sympathetic dystrophy

Inability to bear weight after the injury usually indicates a severe ligament injury or a fracture. A history of 'popping' may suggest injury to the peroneal tendons or a ligament avulsion injury or rupture.

Predisposing factors include:
- walking or running on uneven ground
- wearing inappropriate footwear with little support
- peroneal muscle weakness
- inflexibility of the gastrocnemius–soleus complex
- poor proprioception.

Examination
The extent and site of swelling and ecchymosis, which is more extensive in severe injuries, should be assessed. Palpate each ligament for local tenderness: point bony tenderness is a fracture until proven otherwise. The anterior drawer test (Figure 4.2) and talar tilt (Figure 4.3) to check the anterior talofibular ligament, calcaneofibular ligament and possibly the posterior talofibular ligament should be used to assess stability. Syndesmosis injuries cause tenderness in the anterior lower leg and ankle, which increases with squeezing the fibula against the tibia and with passive ankle dorsiflexion with eversion of the foot. Evaluation of peroneal tendon

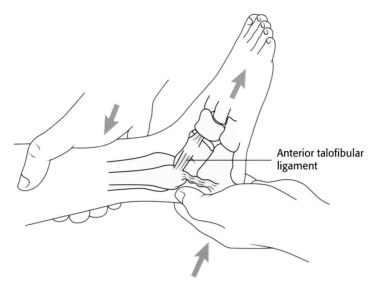

Anterior talofibular
ligament

Figure 4.2 The anterior drawer test, which is used to check the integrity of the anterior talofibular ligament. The patient is supine with his relaxed foot and ankle over the edge of the couch. With one hand, the examiner stabilizes the lower leg and with the other hand holds the patient's foot in 20° of plantar flexion and draws the talus forward in the ankle mortise. Excessive translation (particularly with no firm end-point) in comparison to the contralateral side is a positive test.

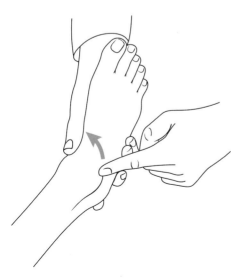

Figure 4.3 The talar tilt test. The patient is supine with the knee in flexion (to relax the gastrocnemius). The talus is tilted into adduction by the examiner. Feel for any opening up of the lateral side of the ankle. Compare range of tilt with the contralateral side.

43

function, neurovascular status and a proprioceptive assessment is also mandatory.

The Ottawa ankle rules are used by many as guidance on the necessity for an X-ray of the ankle and foot after an ankle or foot injury, and are described in Table 4.2.

Management

Ankle sprains must be taken seriously. A poorly managed sprain can result in permanent disability. Most grade III injuries (see Table 2.3, page 21) can usually be treated conservatively but surgical repair may be needed. Exclusion of a diastasis of the tibiofibular joint is essential.

Acute phase. At 0–72 hours, use the PRICES-MM regimen (see page 31), and begin range-of-motion exercises.

TABLE 4.2

The Ottawa ankle rules: when to use ankle or foot radiography*

Ankle injury

Standard radiograph of the ankle is indicated if the patient has pain near the malleoli and one or more of the following:

- Age ≥ 55 years
- Inability to bear weight
- Bone tenderness at the posterior edge or tip of either malleolus

Foot injury

Standard radiograph of the foot is indicated if the patient has pain in the midfoot and one or more of the following:

- Bone tenderness at the:
  - navicular bone
  - cuboid
  - base of the fifth metatarsal
- Inability to bear weight

*From Stiell et al. 1994

Subacute and final stages. Address the causative factors. Begin light load bearing as early as possible in this stage. Flexibility and muscle-strengthening exercises and proprioceptive training are imperative. The analgesic and anti-inflammatory measures used in the acute phase may be helpful during rehabilitation. An ankle support may be helpful, but probably only by providing proprioceptive feedback. It is not a substitute for rehabilitation.

Return to sporting activities should not be attempted without completing a thorough rehabilitation programme and regaining balance, strength and speed.

The causes of chronic ankle pain and dysfunction following acute or repeated ankle sprain are numerous (see Table 4.1). Careful evaluation is imperative and imaging using bone scintigraphy, CT or MRI may be required.

CHAPTER 5
Achilles tendinopathies

Achilles tendinopathies encompass a range of disorders, including inflammation of the paratenon (*paratenonitis*), core degeneration of the tendon substance (*tendinosis*), and a combination of inflammation and degeneration of the tendon with or without a tear (*tendinitis with or without a tear*). Spontaneous ruptures often occur in those patients with asymptomatic intratendinous degeneration. *Insertional tendinitis* is an inflammatory condition at the insertion of the tendon onto the calcaneus (i.e. it is an enthesopathy). It may be associated with a Haglund's deformity (see page 50) and retrocalcaneal and/or retroachilles bursae. The Achilles tendon and related disorders are shown in Figure 5.1.

Clinical features
Symptoms can vary from pain, stiffness and severe inflammation to a minor ache (Table 5.1). Pain may be worst at the beginning of the day, and patients may find it difficult to put their foot to the floor when getting out of bed. Precipitating factors must be sought, and the patient should be questioned about their activities, type of footwear and any trauma.

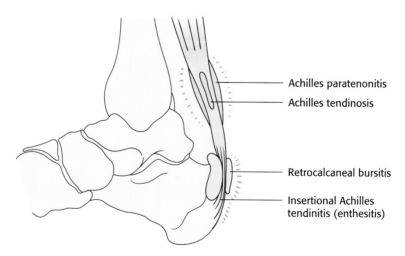

Achilles paratenonitis
Achilles tendinosis

Retrocalcaneal bursitis

Insertional Achilles
tendinitis (enthesitis)

Figure 5.1 The Achilles tendon and related disorders.

TABLE 5.1

Achilles tendinopathies

Condition	Clinical features
Paratenonitis	• Pain and tenderness along Achilles tendon sheath • Inflammation evident, with crepitus and 'creaking' of the tendon
Tendinosis	• May be asymptomatic • Pain varies • Tender Achilles tendon, often with fusiform thickening • Nodule may be palpable
Tendinitis	• Pain and variable inflammation of the tendon • Tender Achilles tendon, often with fusiform thickening • Nodule may be present
Rupture	• Pain • Swelling • Dysfunction • Palpable gap • Altered 'angle of dangle' (see Figure 5.2) • Positive Thomson's test
Enthesitis	• Pain • Inflammation and tenderness at Achilles insertion • May be associated with retrocalcaneal bursitis • Look for Haglund's deformity on X-ray
Retrocalcaneal bursitis	• Pain anterior to the tendon, demonstrated by squeezing the area with two fingers • Look for Haglund's deformity on X-ray

In the sporting population, a careful history must be taken of training patterns, surfaces, equipment use (including shoes), previous injuries and additional training activities (Table 5.2). In individuals with insertional tendinopathies, it is important to explore the possibility of an associated spondyloarthritis (Table 2.5, page 24).

TABLE 5.2

Factors predisposing to Achilles tendinopathies in runners*

Extrinsic factors

- Overtraining (too much/too soon/too often)
- Training type, e.g. too much heavy-weight training involving the calves
- Inappropriate surface
- Poor footwear (too old, poor cushioning, high heel tab, wrong size)
- Poor technique
- Environment (usually extreme cold)
- Drugs: fluoroquinolone antibiotics, anabolic steroids

Intrinsic factors

- Biomechanical malalignments, including gait abnormalities (usually hyperpronation)
- Stiff gastrocnemius–soleus complex, tight hamstrings
- Leg length discrepancy
- Muscle imbalance
- Hyper- or hypomobile hindfoot
- Haglund's deformity
- Spondyloarthritides (enthesopathies)

*Most of these factors apply to many lower-limb soft tissue injuries in sport. Some can be extrapolated to the general population

Examination

Paratenonitis, tendinosis, tendinitis and tears most commonly occur in the mid-third of the tendon, where the area is relatively hypovascular. Local tenderness, inflammatory signs and/or a palpable tendon nodule may be evident. Stiffness of the gastrocnemius–soleus complex is common and can be a major factor limiting progress with rehabilitation if not addressed early.

Complete tears of the Achilles tendon can be diagnosed by assessing the 'angle of dangle' of the feet over the end of the examining couch (Figure 5.2). Diagnosis is confirmed by an absence of plantar flexion of

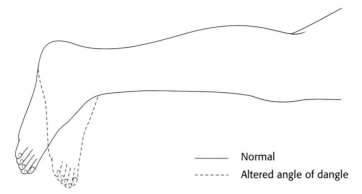

_____ Normal

- - - - - - Altered angle of dangle

Figure 5.2 Complete tears of the Achilles tendon can be diagnosed by assessing the 'angle of dangle' of the feet over the end of the examining couch.

the foot on squeezing the calf (Thomson's test, see Figure 5.3). A palpable gap may be present.

Acute spontaneous ruptures. The history of a loud 'bang' and a feeling as if the patient has been kicked in the back of the leg is virtually diagnostic.

Partial tears of the Achilles tendon may result from a distinct episode or a series of episodes. They are often difficult to diagnose; weakness of plantar

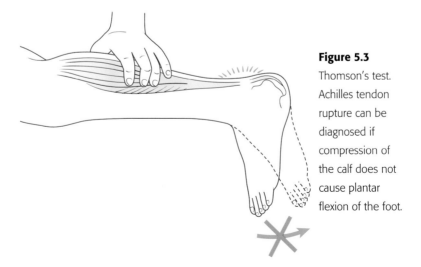

Figure 5.3
Thomson's test.
Achilles tendon
rupture can be
diagnosed if
compression of
the calf does not
cause plantar
flexion of the foot.

flexion, a failure to respond to conservative management and very localized tenderness should arouse suspicion.

Insertional tendinitis can be associated with a Haglund's deformity. This is an abnormal projection of the posterosuperior aspect of the calcaneus and can be caused by recurrent friction, particularly in association with a hypermobile and/or varus rearfoot. A round bony swelling may be evident at the posterosuperior aspect of the calcaneus or just lateral to the Achilles insertion. Radiographic evaluation confirms the presence of the deformity and can be helpful in determining the degree of prominence of the projection.

Haglund's syndrome consists of a retrocalcaneal bursitis in the presence of this deformity and presents with posterior heel pain, which worsens on dorsiflexion of the ankle. Bursal distension, with a tender swelling bulging at both sides of the tendon, may be present.

Other considerations. Gait should be assessed for hyperpronation, leg-length discrepancy and deformities. Always examine the patient's footwear closely and inspect the:
- heel tabs
- heel counter
- midsole
- wear pattern of the sole (which may indicate a hyperpronatory gait)
- overall condition and suitability for the purpose for which it is being worn.

Imaging
MRI and ultrasound are the two most useful means of imaging the Achilles tendon and surrounding structures (Figure 5.4). Both can show areas of degeneration within the tendon and areas of inflammation in either the tendon 'sheath' or the tendon itself. Retrocalcaneal and retroachilles bursae are also detected using these imaging modalities. The reported sensitivity to the detection of tears is variable, but these techniques remain the best approach.

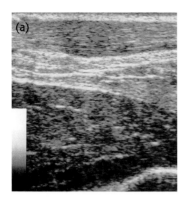 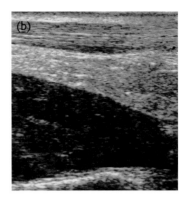

Figure 5.4 Saggital ultrasound images of the (a) left and (b) right Achilles tendons showing an increase in the anteroposterior diameter of the left Achilles tendon (arrow) compared with the right. These are early signs of tendinosis. Note at present that the fibrillar pattern remains well defined and there is no evidence of developing cystic degeneration.

Management

Non-surgical management is appropriate for most cases. Counselling is vital: the patient must be warned that progress may be very slow. Initially, the PRICES-MM approach (see page 31) is appropriate. Rest is relative; alternative modes of activity that do not stress the tendon (swimming, cycling) are permitted. Whilst heel raises may be useful, they should not be worn constantly. When the very acute symptoms have resolved, early, isolated stretching of the gastrocnemius and soleus muscles and hamstrings is very important.

Local modalities including ultrasound, deep heat and laser may be useful. Massage often confers benefit, as can the use of a dorsiflexed night splint. Functional orthoses should be considered. Gradual strength training of the lower leg musculature should be introduced when the patient is pain free. Eccentric loading is particularly effective in regaining strength.

Attention to precipitating factors is very important. This may include altering training in terms of intensity, types of surfaces, addressing errors in technique and changing equipment, particularly footwear, as discussed above. Heel tabs should be cut down to avoid impingement on the tendon. In those individuals with Haglund's deformity, padding may be useful over the exostosis.

Corticosteroid injections have no role as they are usually ineffective and may weaken the tendon with resulting rupture, although some advocate their use in paratenonitis.

Return to activity should be gradual and monitored closely. The key to success is ensuring that the patient has a full understanding of the disorder and that the process of recovery may be lengthy.

Surgical intervention should be reserved for those few who fail to respond to conservative management and those with total ruptures or significant partial tears. Some surgeons advocate a tendon-splitting procedure in cases of chronic Achilles tendinitis.

Patients with an Achilles tendinopathy (often insertional) and/or a retrocalcaneal bursitis in association with a Haglund's deformity and who fail to respond to non-surgical measures require surgical excision of the offending areas of bone. In some cases of chronic tendinopathy, excision of an area of focal degeneration may be needed.

CHAPTER 6

Plantar fasciitis

True plantar fasciitis is an inflammatory disorder of the plantar fascia at its origin on the base of the calcaneus (Figure 6.1). However, the term is commonly used to describe any pain (inflammatory or non-inflammatory) in the plantar fascia.

As it pronates, the foot is lengthened by flattening of the medial arch, with resulting tension on the plantar fascial origin. This traction may lead to inflammation at the origin. Irritation of the periosteum can result in new bone formation and a traction spur. Such spurs are a result, not the cause, of the injury and are frequently found in asymptomatic individuals. The injury may lead to tightening of the plantar fascia, which can be worsened by further overuse. Treatment aims to reduce the tension in the fascia.

(a)

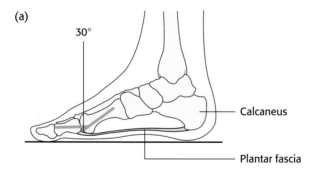

(b)

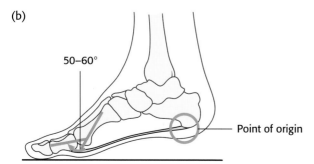

Figure 6.1 The plantar fascia. (a) When the whole foot is loaded and (b) during toe-off, when the fascia is stretched.

Patients may seek advice at the later stages of the complaint, when inflammation is less of a feature, but cyclical, chronic pain, partly due to tightness of the fascia, may be more prominent. Factors predisposing to plantar fasciitis are listed in Table 6.1.

Clinical features

Patients present with pain in the plantar or plantar-medial aspect of the calcaneus, where the intrinsic muscles of the foot and the fascia itself insert into the base of the calcaneus. Onset of pain may be gradual or acute. Pain and stiffness in the plantar tissues are most noticeable in the morning. Placing the foot on the floor on rising from bed is often excruciating, and results from stretching the tight (and often inflamed) fascia; the discomfort tends to ease after a few steps. Weight-bearing activity, particularly in poorly cushioned unsupportive footwear, exacerbates the symptoms.

Differential diagnosis. Point tenderness of the calcaneus at the origin of the plantar fascia and pain exacerbated with passive stretching of the fascia may be present with plantar fasciitis. However, there are other causes of pain as outlined in Table 6.2. With a 'bruised heel', the pain is under the entire weight-bearing surface of the calcaneus and an atrophic fat pad may be evident. Symptoms may be acute after a traumatic episode (a long walk or run) to which the patient is unused, although such a history may also be given with plantar fasciitis.

TABLE 6.1

Factors predisposing to plantar fasciitis

- Obesity
- Pes cavus
- Pes planus, over-pronation
- Wearing inappropriate footwear, e.g. hard boots, flexible midsole, poor heel counter
- High activity levels on hard surfaces, e.g. distance running on roads
- Disease, e.g. diabetes, spondyloarthritis

TABLE 6.2

Differential diagnosis of plantar heel pain

- Plantar fasciitis/plantar fascial pain
- Heel fat pad syndrome/bruised heel
- Stress fracture of calcaneus
- Entrapment of the medial calcaneal branch of the posterior tibial nerve
- Inflammatory arthropathy
- Referred from back, particularly when heel pain is bilateral

Treatment

In the acute phase, ice, relative rest, supportive taping, a heel cup (often more helpful for heel fat pad syndrome), analgesics or NSAIDs may be beneficial. Physiotherapists may use ultrasound or laser therapy although their effects are as yet unproven. Taping is effective for relieving pain and helps to confirm the diagnosis of plantar fasciitis as it is usually ineffective for the other differential diagnoses. Taping should only be used in the acute phase since stretching of the plantar fascia and gastrocnemius–soleus complex is vital. Night splints can be very effective, although compliance is reported to be poor. An orthotic is often helpful.

Treatment may be prolonged. In resistant cases other diagnoses, particularly stress fractures, need to be excluded.

Local corticosteroid (hydrocortisone) administration should be restricted to those patients who have point tenderness at the origin on the calcaneus and who have failed to respond to conservative measures.

Surgery (release of the plantar fascia) is rarely indicated and is reserved for those few who continue to have severe symptoms. In chronic cases, correction of predisposing factors is usually necessary.

CHAPTER 7
Lateral epicondylitis (tennis elbow)

Lateral epicondylitis is a common condition. It results from repetitive movements of the hand and forearm that cause injury to the tendon of the extensor supinator muscle group (Figure 7.1). Extensor carpi radialis brevis is most frequently involved. It affects not only up to 40% of tennis players, but a wide range of individuals, including carpenters and musicians, and more commonly affects the dominant arm. It is particularly prevalent among those aged 40–60 years, and is estimated to affect 1–4% of the population.

Clinical features
The history is usually that of chronic overuse of forearm musculature, although the condition can arise after a single episode of local trauma. Pain in the lateral aspect of the forearm, near the lateral epicondyle, particularly during grip is a feature and simple daily tasks may become difficult.

On examination, there is local tenderness at the lateral epicondyle, with pain on passive wrist flexion (particularly with the elbow in extension; Figure 7.2) and with resisted wrist and middle finger extension. Grip strength is limited by pain at the lateral epicondyle. Other causes, such

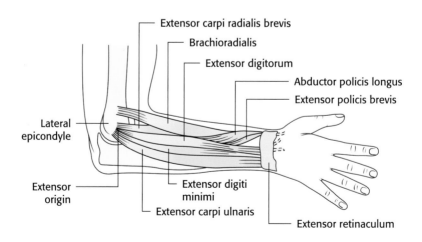

Figure 7.1 Lateral epicondyle anatomy, showing the extensor supinator muscle group.

(a)

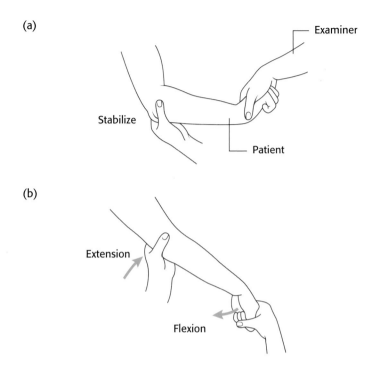

(b)

Figure 7.2 The tennis elbow test. (a) Method 1. The patient makes a fist, pronates the forearm then radially deviates and extends the wrist against the examiner's resistance. (b) Method 2. The examiner pronates the patient's forearm, flexes the wrist fully and extends the elbow. In both, a positive test is indicated by pain at the lateral epicondyle.

as referred pain, need to be considered if specific provocation tests for epicondylitis are negative. Other causes of lateral elbow pain are listed in Table 7.1.

Precipitating causes. It is of paramount importance to address the precipitating causes of the injury. In occupational situations, repeated performance of tasks that are ergonomically difficult or stressful on the forearm is common. The introduction of frequent, regular rest periods at work may be enough to prevent recurrence. Aetiological factors in the sporting situation for a true 'tennis elbow' are listed in Table 7.2, and these can be extrapolated to most situations. Failure to address these issues is likely to result in failure to respond to therapy or recurrence of the problem.

TABLE 7.1

Differential diagnosis of lateral elbow pain

- Lateral epicondylitis
- Extensor myalgia
- Radial (posterior interosseous) nerve entrapment
- C6 root lesion
- Brachialgia
- Osteochondritis dissecans
- Osteochondrosis of the radiocapitellar joint
- Instability of the radiocapitellar joint
- Bursitis at the radial head
- Bony tumour

Treatment

Relative rest is vital. In severe cases, a cock-up wrist support, which may be worn at night, may relieve the tension on the common extensor insertion. Local ice and the use of other modalities such as laser, ultrasound and deep heat may help. Support with an adjustable compression strap applied to the proximal forearm helps to prevent full contraction of the extensor muscle group during work. Gradual stretching is important.

NSAIDs. Oral NSAIDs are commonly prescribed, but topical anti-inflammatory gels are safer and may provide more effective relief.

Corticosteroid injections to the peritendinous area just off the bone are often used unnecessarily and should be reserved for resistant cases. Short-acting preparations such as hydrocortisone should be used and injection guidelines followed closely. There is some evidence that dry needling of the area is as beneficial as corticosteroid injections. Acupuncture may also be used for pain control.

Exercise. Stretching of the forearm extensors needs to commence early. A progressive exercise regimen to strengthen the wrist and finger extensors

TABLE 7.2

True tennis elbow: precipitating causes

General

- Inadequate conditioning/muscle weakness
- Lack of warm up
- Lack of stretching
- Inadequate rest periods between matches/training sessions
- Overuse

Equipment

- Has the patient changed equipment recently?
- Tennis racquet grip too large/small
- Racquet too heavy/light
- Racquet too stiff (particularly new compounds)
- String tension too tight/loose
- Court surface too fast
- Tennis balls too heavy/wet

Technique

- Too much grip tension
- Elbow leading in backhand
- Snapping wrist in backhand
- Awkward body movement in stroke (use body and shoulder rotation)
- Poor energy transfer from lower trunk

should be introduced gradually, but with caution as it may aggravate the condition.

Surgery. If full conservative measures prove unsuccessful, surgical intervention may be necessary. Some of the tissues around the lateral epicondyle can be released, areas of mucoid degeneration excised or a synovial fringe can be removed from the radiohumeral joint if necessary.

CHAPTER 8
Shoulder disorders

More than 90% of episodes of shoulder pain are due to non-articular causes, the two most common disorders being rotator cuff lesions and adhesive capsulitis (frozen shoulder). The anatomy of the shoulder complex and sites of shoulder pain are shown in Figures 8.1–8.3, while the differential diagnoses of shoulder pain are listed in Table 8.1.

General clinical features

These are presented in Tables 8.2 and 8.3. The patient's age may give a clue to diagnosis. Instability should be suspected in the younger patient under 25 years of age. Degenerative cuff tears are unusual in people aged under 40 years. Adhesive capsulitis occurs in those aged over 40 years.

Rotator cuff tendinitis

The rotator cuff confers up to 50% of the power of the shoulder in abduction and 80% in external rotation (Table 8.4). It also stabilizes the humeral head in the glenoid. Rotator cuff tendinopathies include inflammatory and degenerative lesions and/or partial or complete tears of

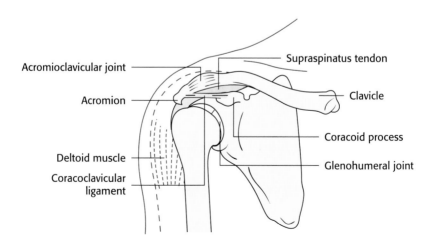

Figure 8.1 The functional anatomy of the shoulder complex.

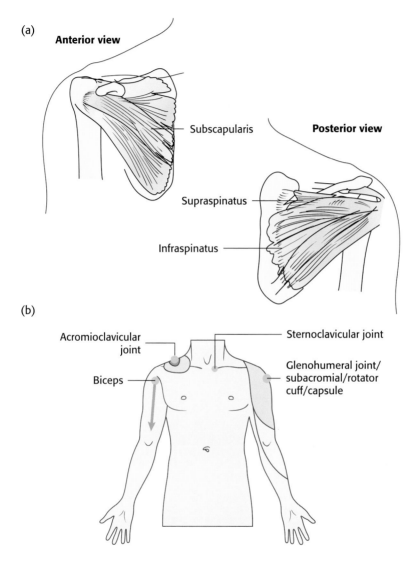

Figure 8.2 (a) The muscles of the rotator cuff. (b) Sites of pain.

one or more tendons of the rotator cuff. Impingement on the cuff can occur in relation to several factors (Table 8.5).

Clinical features. The presenting symptom is usually pain in the lateral aspect of the upper arm. A history of recent trauma or overuse may be

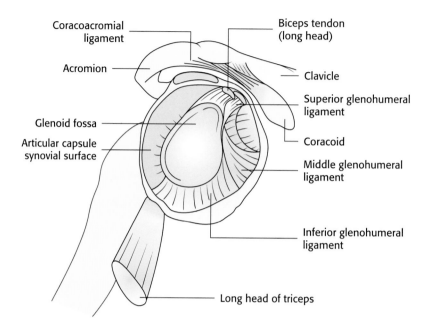

Coracoacromial ligament

Biceps tendon (long head)

Acromion

Clavicle

Superior glenohumeral ligament

Glenoid fossa

Articular capsule synovial surface

Coracoid

Middle glenohumeral ligament

Inferior glenohumeral ligament

Long head of triceps

Figure 8.3 The rim of the glenoid is lined with a fibrocartilaginous rim called the glenoid labrum that surrounds the shallow glenoid fossa and deepens the fossa to allow greater stability of the humeral head.

given, particularly by younger individuals in whom instability of the joint often plays an important role. In the minority of such cases, there may be a history of subluxation or dislocation. Alternatively, particularly in older patients, pain may increase gradually. Pain when performing overhead activities may occur, particularly if impingement is a factor. Pain at night when lying on the affected side or turning over in bed is common. Carrying heavy objects may be difficult due to pain or weakness. Clicking may be noted with glenohumeral instability or tendinitis, the latter particularly where the biceps is involved.

Some cases of rotator cuff tendinitis are associated with calcific deposits, which are evident on X-ray. In many cases, the finding may be coincidental; in others, there may be an acute onset of severe tendinitis, with systemic symptoms ('calcific tendinitis'). The cause of the calcium deposition is unknown. In most cases, the calcium will be resorbed and the symptoms will gradually settle.

TABLE 8.1

Differential diagnosis of shoulder pain*

- Rotator cuff tendinopathy ± impingement
- Rotator cuff tear
- Subacromial bursitis
- Frozen shoulder (capsulitis)
- Glenohumeral pathology**
- Acromioclavicular pathology**
- Sternocostal pathology**
- Glenoid labral lesions
- Referred pain (from neck, intrathoracic, subdiaphragmatic lesions)
- Systemic disease, such as polymyalgia rheumatica
- Rare causes, such as thoracic outlet syndrome
- Myofascial pain syndromes

*Conditions may coexist
**Arthritis, instability, sepsis, neoplasm

Examination may reveal wasting of the muscles of the cuff; this is usually associated with a cuff tear or disuse after very severe tendinitis. Pseudo-winging may occur as a result. Active movements may be limited by pain and a painful arc may be present. Profound weakness of abduction or an inability to maintain the arm in 90° of abduction suggests a massive rotator cuff tear, but full active movement is frequently maintained in the presence of a full-thickness cuff tear. Passive movements should be full, but pain from impingement often makes this difficult. Significant pain with resisted testing of different portions of the cuff may indicate the site of a rotator cuff tendinopathy. Weakness out of proportion to pain indicates that a tear is present. Testing for impingement is important (Figure 8.4).

Testing for instability should be undertaken, and is particularly important in the younger and/or sporting patient. Inferior laxity, which usually indicates multidirectional laxity, may be demonstrated by the inferior sulcus sign (Figure 8.5). When anterior or posterior instability is present, the

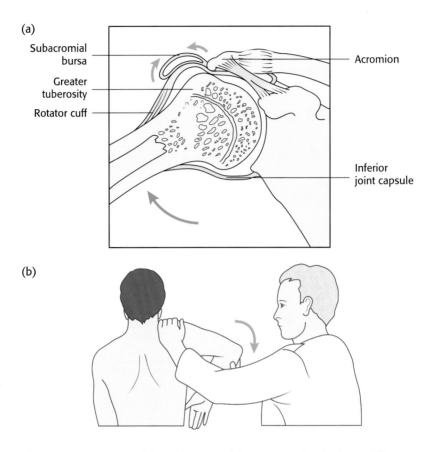

Figure 8.4 Impingement. (a) Impingement of the rotator cuff and subacromial bursa between the coracoacromial arch and the humeral head. (b) With the patient standing with the examiner passively abducting the affected arm to 90° abduction and 30° forward flexion, the examiner then passively internally rotates the arm. The patient will complain of pain in the presence of impingement.

patient becomes apprehensive that the shoulder may be about to come out of joint when performing the appropriate apprehension tests (Figure 8.6). In cases of occult instability or generalized joint laxity, these tests may or may not elicit pain but with no apprehension.

Imaging is often unnecessary. Plain radiographs (anteroposterior and axial views) may show subacromial osteophytes, if present, and the anatomy of the subacromial space. Anatomical factors that may predispose to the condition, such as a shallow subacromial space and a hooked acromion, may be evident.

Both ultrasound and MRI can be used effectively to demonstrate rotator cuff tendinitis and partial- and full-thickness tears (Figure 8.7). They are not entirely conclusive. Patients who fail to respond to conservative therapy or have evidence of a significant rotator cuff tear warrant MRI or ultrasound imaging to look for a tear. An arthrogram may be required if other imaging measures fail to confirm a strong suspicion of a full-thickness tear.

Management of rotator cuff tendinopathies. Relative rest of the affected arm is necessary. In the acute phase, ice, simple analgesics, NSAIDs, acupuncture and laser therapy may help. If early benefit is not gained with NSAIDs, they should not be continued. Later, deep heat, laser, ultrasound and massage may all be used by the physiotherapist and a gradual regimen of stretching and cuff strengthening exercises, including a muscle balance and re-education programme for those patients with instability, can be introduced. Factors such as posture, capsular or thoracic stiffness and scapular stability need to be addressed.

Attention to the precipitating and contributing factors is important. This includes introducing rest periods at work in those patients who are performing repetitive overhead tasks.

Corticosteroids. In patients with tendinopathies in the absence of clinical evidence of a tear, subacromial corticosteroid injections may be administered. However, these should be reserved for those cases that do not settle with the above measures. Injections should follow the usual guidelines. They are rarely required in the young patient.

Surgery should be reserved for active patients with a rotator cuff rupture (almost universally occurring subsequent to trauma in this group), those with a significant post-traumatic tear or those with a tear or tendinitis that fail to respond to non-surgical management. Surgery for these patients may involve subacromial decompression with or without repair of the tear. There is some suggestion that early surgery may be appropriate for patients with a rotator cuff tear and a rupture of the long head of the biceps, as they are more likely to develop rotator cuff arthropathy.

TABLE 8.2

Shoulder disorders: patient characteristics and symptoms

Disorder	Age (years)	Onset	Trauma	Pain site
Rotator cuff tendinitis	Any	Acute/chronic	±	S/RC
Calcific tendinitis	30–60	Acute	–	S/RC
Partial-thickness rotator cuff tear	• Acute: any • Chronic: particularly > 40	Acute/chronic	May be trivial in older patients	S/RC
Full-thickness rotator cuff tear	Particularly affects those > 40	Acute/chronic	• Severe in young patients • May be trivial in older patients	S/RC
Subacromial bursitis	Any	Acute/chronic	±	S/RC
Glenohumeral joint instability	< 30	Episodic	Possible	S/RC
Labral tear	< 40	Acute/chronic	+	S/RC

*True weakness, but note that all disorders can cause weakness in association with pain
–, absent → ++++, extreme

Night pain	Clicking	Weakness*	Instability	Associations
++	+ (particularly in younger patients with instability)	±	± (particularly in younger patients)	• Instability in young patients • Degeneration in older patients • Impingement
+++	±	–	–	• ?Cuff degeneration
+++	+	++	± in younger patients	• Instability and/or trauma in young patients • Degeneration in older patients
+++	+	++++ (depending on size of tear)	–	• > 40 years: degenerative cuff • > 40 years: after dislocation
++	±	–	±	• Impingement
–	±	In acute episodes	++	• Rotator cuff + biceps pathologies • Muscle imbalance • Hypermobility • Neurological symptoms in acute episodes
–	++ Clunking	–	+	• Instability • Throwing sports

S/RC, shoulder/rotator cuff; B, biceps tendon; ACJ, acromioclavicular joint; sscap, suprascapular; see Figure 8.2b, page 61

TABLE 8.2 (continued)

Disorder	Age (years)	Onset	Trauma	Pain site
Rupture of long head of biceps	> 40	Acute/insidious	±	B S/RC Often nil
Bicipital tendinitis	Any	Acute/chronic	−	B S/RC
Frozen shoulder	40–70	Acute/subacute/ chronic	±	S/RC
ACJ osteoarthritis	> 30	Chronic	−	ACJ
ACJ sprain	Any	Acute	++	ACJ
Glenohumeral joint arthropathy	> 40	Chronic	−	S/RC
Cervical spondylosis	> 35	Chronic	±	sscap

*True weakness, but note that all disorders can cause weakness in association with pain
−, absent → ++++, extreme

Glenoid labrum injuries

Pathology of the glenoid labrum can occur particularly in individuals
with some degree of instability of the shoulder joint after trauma.
Such labral injuries include SLAP (superior labral anterior posterior
tear) lesions. Clinical evaluation often reveals symptoms and
signs suggestive of rotator cuff and bicipital tendinopathies, with
additional features such as catching and snapping of the shoulder
on internal rotation of the arm. CT or MRI arthrography may
help to confirm the lesion, but diagnosis is often made only at
arthroscopy.

Management is primarily surgical and usually arthroscopic.

Night pain	Clicking	Weakness*	Instability	Associations
±	+	±	–	• Rotator cuff disease
±	+	–	±	• Majority associated with instability or rotator cuff disease
+++	–	–	–	• See pages 73–6
++	++	–	–	• May cause cuff pathology
++	++	–	+	• Trauma
+	++	– (crepitus)	–	–
±	±	+	–	• Neurological symptoms

S/RC, shoulder/rotator cuff; B, biceps tendon; ACJ, acromioclavicular joint; sscap, suprascapular; see Figure 8.2b, page 61

Adhesive capsulitis

The frozen shoulder is one of the most common causes of shoulder pain and disability seen by physicians, affecting 2–3% of the non-diabetic population. Those most commonly affected are aged between 40 and 70 years; women are slightly more prone to frozen shoulder than men.

Pathophysiology. This is poorly understood as available reports tend to represent late-stage disease. Macroscopically, the capsule is thickened and contracted. Infiltration of the subsynovial capsule by chronic inflammatory cells, fibrosis and focal degeneration of collagen have been described. However, these changes are non-specific and have been seen on autopsy in

69

TABLE 8.3

Shoulder disorders: clinical signs

Disorder	Wasting	Painful arc	Active range of movement	Passive range of movement
Rotator cuff tendinitis	±	+++	Limited by pain only	Full*
Calcific tendinitis	±	++	Limited by pain only	Full*
Partial-thickness rotator cuff tear	+	++	May be reduced	Full*
Full-thickness rotator cuff tear	++	+	↓↓↓	Full (↓ late)
Subacromial bursitis	–	++	Limited by pain only	Full*
GHJ instability	–	±	Normal	Normal
Labral tear	–	±	Normal	Normal
Rupture of long head of biceps	–	–	Normal	Full
Bicipital tendinitis	–	±	Normal	Full
Frozen shoulder	±	+ (early)	Global ↓↓↓	Global ↓
ACJ osteoarthritis	–	Superior arc	↓ full elevation	May be ↓↓ full elevation
ACJ sprain	–	± superior arc	↓ full elevation	Full*
GHJ arthropathy	±	–	↓	↓
Cervical spondylosis	–	–	Normal	Normal

*May be limited by patient's pain
**The planes in which pain and/or weakness are noted indicates the portion(s) of the cuff involved
GHJ, glenohumeral joint; ACJ, acromioclavicular joint

Resisted tests	Impingement	Instability	Others
Pain > weakness**	+++	−	−
Pain > weakness**	+++	−	+++ Local tenderness
Pain and weakness (may vary)	++/−	−	−
Weakness >> pain	++	−	−
± Pain	++	−	−
Normal	±	+++	Positive apprehension test(s)
Normal	±	++	−
• Often normal • ± Weakness of elbow • ± Shoulder flexion • ± Forearm supination only‡	± (may be present with concurrent rotator cuff tendinitis)	−	Visible deformity
Pain on forward flexion of a straight arm	−	±	Provocation tests
Normal	+ (early)	−	See pages 73–6
Normal	−	−	• ± Local deformity • Tenderness ++ • Positive ACJ stress test • Radiological changes
Normal	−	−	• ± Local deformity • Tenderness ++ • Positive ACJ stress test • Positive stress films
Normal	−	−	Radiological changes
Normal	−	−	↓/Painful neck movements

‡Weakness of supination indicates rupture of radial (distal) insertion of biceps tendon: surgical intervention is necessary in such cases
−, absent → +++, marked

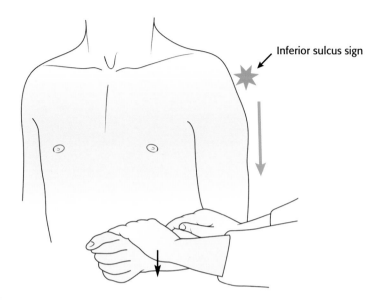

Inferior sulcus sign

Figure 8.5 The inferior sulcus sign, which occurs on downward traction on the arm.

TABLE 8.4

Main actions of the rotator cuff

Muscles*	Action
Supraspinatus	Initiation of abduction but active throughout range
Subscapularis	Internal rotation
Infraspinatus	External rotation
Teres minor	External rotation
Biceps (not formally part of the rotator cuff, but closely associated with it)	Elbow flexion; forearm supination; also acts as a stabilizer

*All act to stabilize the humeral head in the glenoid fossa during movement

TABLE 8.5

Causes of rotator cuff tendinopathies

Primary inflammation

- Macrotrauma
- Microtrauma (repetitive overuse)
- Calcification (acute calcific tendinitis)
- Inflammatory arthropathies

Glenohumeral instability

- Dislocation/subluxation
- Inherent joint laxity
- Muscle imbalance/rotator cuff weakness

Impingement

- Static
  - type II or III acromion morphology
  - acromioclavicular osteophytes
  - acromial spur
  - capsulitis
- Dynamic
  - muscle imbalance, cuff weakness
  - instability

Degeneration

- Hypovascularity of the rotator cuff
- Age

normal shoulders. Four stages of pathology have been described from arthroscopic observations (Table 8.6); other investigators have found little evidence of inflammation or even adhesions in this condition.

Clinical features. Frozen shoulder can occur spontaneously or after trauma or illness (Table 8.7). Diagnosis should be made on clinical grounds, although ultrasound or arthrography can be helpful (Table 8.8). Patients present with acute, subacute or chronic pain and stiffness in one or both shoulders. Night pain is common. Both passive and active glenohumeral movements are globally restricted in the absence of significant glenohumeral osteoarthritis. The natural history is one of recovery, but this can take 3 years or more. Involvement of the contralateral shoulder occurs in 17% of cases within 5 years. Fifteen per cent of patients have a long-term detectable reduction in glenohumeral movement.

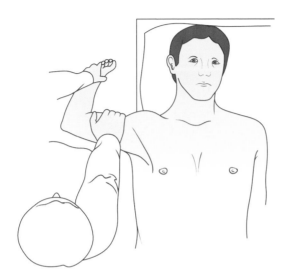

Figure 8.6 The anterior apprehension test. With anterior instability, the patient becomes apprehensive that the shoulder is about to come out of joint.

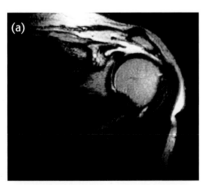

(a)

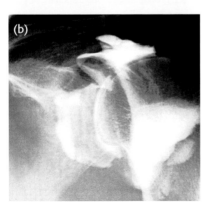

(b)

Figure 8.7 (a) A T2-weighted MR image of the shoulder. Note the position of the torn supraspinatus tendon, the unfavourable acromion and the small gap between the acromion and the humeral head. The high-signal intensity region is fluid. (b) The corresponding arthrographic image shows escape of contrast from the joint, confirming a full-thickness tear of the rotator cuff.

TABLE 8.6

Arthroscopic and clinical features of frozen shoulder*

Stage	Arthroscopic findings	Clinical features
1	• Mild fibrinous synovitis • Inflammatory reaction is detectable, particularly in and around the axillary fold of the joint	• Similar to impingement syndrome
2	• Red, thickened and inflamed synovium • Adhesions can be visualized extending from the dependent fold to the humeral head	• Global restriction of movement, with pain
3	• Synovium less inflamed but the dependent fold is reduced to half its original size	• As above
4	• No evidence of synovitis • Mature adhesions • Humeral head severely compressed against the glenoid and the biceps tendon	• Pain is less of a feature • Restriction continues

*From Nevasier and Nevasier 1987

Management. Pain relief and the restoration of motion and function of the shoulder are the objectives of treatment. Most patients recover with time, and management involves controlling pain and maintaining movement while the condition runs its course. Counselling the patient about the nature and often prolonged course of the condition is imperative.

A wide variety of treatment modalities have been advocated in the management of frozen shoulder, including corticosteroids, physiotherapy, NSAIDs, manipulation under anaesthetic and infiltration brisement. However, no regimen has been consistently successful. Local steroid injections may relieve pain and increase the range of motion in the short

TABLE 8.7

Frozen shoulder: associations

- Rotator cuff tendinopathy
- Myocardial infarction
- Respiratory illness
- Thoracotomy
- Immobility, e.g. with stroke
- Diabetes (often severely affected)
- Thyroid disease
- Algodystrophy (secondary to frozen shoulder)

TABLE 8.8

Arthrographic features of frozen shoulder*

- A reduction of joint volume to < 10 ml
- Obliteration of the subscapular and axillary recesses
- Irregularity of the capsular attachment to the anatomical neck of the humerus

*From Nevasier 1980

term, but no long-term benefits have been found. Systemic corticosteroids may also improve pain and shoulder mobility, but again with no demonstrable improvement in the rate of recovery. There is limited evidence of short-term benefit, with respect to range of motion but not pain, with hydrodistension with corticosteroids versus corticosteroids alone in the management of frozen shoulder. Simple measures and exercises can be useful (Table 8.9).

TABLE 8.9

Advice and home exercises for patients with frozen shoulder

Heat and cold therapy

- Heat (e.g. a hot water bottle), 15–20 minutes, particularly before home exercises; patients with significant rest pain or pain at night should not use heat therapy
- Cold (e.g. ice wrapped in a moist towel), 15–20 minutes, four times daily, particularly for those patients with pain at rest and following home exercises

Home exercises*

- Standing, bend over and hang the affected arm loosely downwards
- Rotate the arm gently in a circular motion, 20 rotations in one direction, then 20 in the other
- Try to increase the size of the circle every day

- Sitting or supine with the knees bent, raise the affected arm, with the elbow straight above your head
- With the opposite (good) arm, push the affected arm slightly further to get an additional stretch
- Hold for 5 seconds, then relax
- Repeat 5 times

- Sitting, raise your arms out to the side to 90°
- Turn your palms upwards and continue raising your arms upwards, as far as you can
- Repeat 5–10 times

- Sitting, keep your elbow of the affected arm at your side (a belt around your trunk and elbow will help this)
- Flex your elbow
- Move your forearm out to the side, so that your forearm rotates outwards

---

- Standing, bring your arm behind your back, as if to reach for your wallet or undo your bra
- To get a further stretch, hold a towel in your hand and pull up on the towel with the opposite hand
- Hold for 10 seconds
- Repeat 10 times

Do all of the above exercises twice daily

*Patients should be warned not to *over*-stretch when doing these exercises, and should discontinue if moderate or severe pain occurs

CHAPTER 9
Polymyalgia rheumatica

Polymyalgia rheumatica (PMR) is a clinical syndrome characterized by proximal muscle pain and stiffness.

Clinical features

Patients usually localize their pain to the muscles of the shoulder and pelvic girdles. Symptoms are usually symmetrical and sudden in onset. Women are twice as likely to be affected as men and the mean age of onset is 70 years; it is rare in patients under 50.

Stiffness is usually the predominant symptom; it is worst after rest and in the morning. Systemic symptoms, such as fever, malaise and weight loss, in addition to low mood, are also common. Pain with movement is noted and nocturnal disturbance commonly occurs.

Examination. Active mobility of the shoulders and hips is restricted by pain and stiffness. Passive movements are full. Although strength and range of motion may be limited by pain, true weakness and restriction do not occur. The presence of synovitis is more indicative of a polymyalgic presentation of inflammatory arthritis. There is often tenderness of involved structures including the muscles, bursae, tendons and capsule.

Differential diagnoses of PMR are extensive and PMR is a diagnosis of exclusion (Tables 9.1 and 9.2). A thorough history, examination and appropriate investigations (Table 9.3) are vital in reaching the correct diagnosis.

A significantly elevated erythrocyte sedimentation rate (ESR) usually occurs, although it may be normal in rare cases. However, ESR is often slightly elevated in healthy elderly people. A normocytic, normochromic anaemia and a mild thrombocytosis may occur. A non-specific polyclonal rise in immunoglobulin is often noted, as is a slight rise in alkaline phosphatase of liver origin.

TABLE 9.1

Differential diagnosis of PMR

- Neoplasm
- Lymphoproliferative disease
- Multiple myeloma
- Inflammatory arthritis
- Osteoarthritis, cervical spondylosis
- Connective tissue disease
- Hypothyroidism
- Myositis
- Myopathy
- Parkinsonism
- Fibromyalgia/regional myofascial pain
- Infection
- Bone disease, e.g. osteomalacia, osteomyelitis
- Functional

TABLE 9.2

Diagnostic criteria for PMR*

- Shoulder and pelvic-girdle pain that is primarily muscular in the absence of true muscle weakness
- Morning stiffness
- Duration of at least 2 months unless treated
- Erythrocyte sedimentation rate > 30 mm/hour or C-reactive protein > 6 μg/ml
- Absence of rheumatoid or inflammatory arthritis or malignant disease
- Absence of objective signs of muscle disease
- Prompt and dramatic response to systemic corticosteroids

*Reproduced from Jones and Hazleman 1981

Temporal arteritis

Temporal arteritis, also known as giant cell arteritis, is a form of vasculitis, a panarteritis with a patchy inflammatory infiltrate, affecting one or both temporal arteries and variably other arteries including the carotids and even the aorta. The diagnostic criteria for temporal arteritis are described in Table 9.4.

TABLE 9.3

Investigations in PMR

- Erythrocyte sedimentation rate (or plasma viscosity, and/or C-reactive protein level)
- Full blood count and white cell differential
- Renal, liver and bone biochemistry
- Immunoglobulins and serum electrophoresis
- Urinary Bence-Jones proteins
- Thyroid function
- Creatine kinase
- Rheumatoid factor, autoantibodies*
- Chest X-ray*
- Infection screen*

*Optional, as indicated

Clinical findings relate to the arteries involved. Typically, persistent, severe temporal headache (often bilateral), jaw claudication and scalp tenderness with or without polymyalgia are cardinal features of temporal arteritis. Blindness is the most serious complication, and a history of visual disturbance requires urgent intervention with steroid therapy.

TABLE 9.4

Diagnostic criteria for temporal arteritis*

- Positive temporal artery biopsy or cranial artery tenderness noted by a physician
- One or more of: visual disturbance, headache, jaw pain, cerebrovascular insufficiency
- Erythrocyte sedimentation rate > 30 mm/hour or C-reactive protein > 6 µg/ml
- Response to systemic corticosteroids

*Reproduced from Jones and Hazleman 1981

Temporal artery biopsy is necessary if either the diagnosis is in doubt or the means are readily available without causing a delay in treatment. A negative biopsy does not exclude the diagnosis.

Temporal arteritis and PMR are considered to be closely related, forming a spectrum of the same disorder. Up to 15% of patients with PMR with no symptoms of temporal arteritis have positive temporal artery biopsies.

Management of PMR

A rapid response to systemic steroid therapy (80% improvement within 48 hours) is frequently included in the diagnostic criteria of PMR. If no such significant response to adequate doses occurs, the diagnosis should be reviewed. The ESR usually falls to normal within 2–3 weeks, the C-reactive protein level within 1 week. Progress on treatment is assessed predominantly on symptom relief, as the ESR can be misleading.

The steroid regimen varies according to the individual response. However, an initial dose of 15–20 mg is recommended for the first month and the dose is tapered thereafter (Figure 9.1). Treatment is often prolonged; only one-third to one-half of patients have discontinued steroids after 2 years. Bone prophylaxis in the form of a bisphosphonate is recommended. Possible reasons for non-response to steroid therapy are listed in Table 9.5.

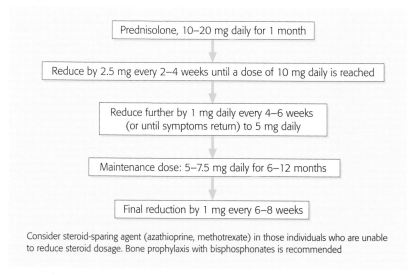

Prednisolone, 10–20 mg daily for 1 month

Reduce by 2.5 mg every 2–4 weeks until a dose of 10 mg daily is reached

Reduce further by 1 mg daily every 4–6 weeks
(or until symptoms return) to 5 mg daily

Maintenance dose: 5–7.5 mg daily for 6–12 months

Final reduction by 1 mg every 6–8 weeks

Consider steroid-sparing agent (azathioprine, methotrexate) in those individuals who are unable to reduce steroid dosage. Bone prophylaxis with bisphosphonates is recommended

Figure 9.1 Treatment regimen for PMR.

TABLE 9.5

Causes for failure to respond to steroid therapy in PMR

- Inadequate steroid dose
- Steroid-resistant disease
- Steroid dose reduced too rapidly
- Incorrect diagnosis
- Additional underlying systemic disorder, e.g. neoplasm

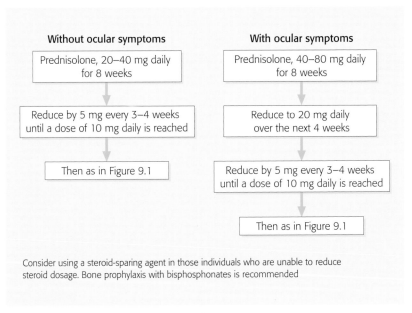

Without ocular symptoms

Prednisolone, 20–40 mg daily
for 8 weeks

↓

Reduce by 5 mg every 3–4 weeks
until a dose of 10 mg daily is reached

↓

Then as in Figure 9.1

With ocular symptoms

Prednisolone, 40–80 mg daily
for 8 weeks

↓

Reduce to 20 mg daily
over the next 4 weeks

↓

Reduce by 5 mg every 3–4 weeks
until a dose of 10 mg daily is reached

↓

Then as in Figure 9.1

Consider using a steroid-sparing agent in those individuals who are unable to reduce
steroid dosage. Bone prophylaxis with bisphosphonates is recommended

Figure 9.2 Treatment regimen for temporal arteritis.

Patients with temporal arteritis require higher doses of steroids and of this group, those with visual symptoms require higher doses (Figure 9.2). Patients who are unable to reduce their steroid dose because of disease activity may benefit from the addition of a 'steroid sparer' (azathioprine or methotrexate).

All patients with PMR and temporal arteritis must be thoroughly counselled about their disease and the significance of associated headache and visual disturbance.

CHAPTER 10

Fibromyalgia and regional myofascial pain syndromes

Fibromyalgia

'Fibromyalgia' is a term used to describe diffuse musculoskeletal pain and tender points with no other definable cause, where a tender point is an area of heightened superficial tenderness on palpation. Fatigue is often also prominent (Table 10.1). Characteristic tender points exist (Figure 10.1); however, other areas can be involved. Clinical examination should otherwise be normal.

TABLE 10.1

Features of fibromyalgia*

Cardinal features**

- Chronic (> 3 months) widespread pain
- Tender points

Characteristic features

- Fatigue
- Sleep disturbance
- Stiffness
- Raynaud's syndrome-like symptoms
- Headache
- Paraesthesiae
- Anxiety
- Depression
- Irritable bowel syndrome

*Criteria of the American College of Rheumatology 1990
**Symptoms must have been present for a minimum of 3 months, and should have involved the upper and lower body bilaterally as well as the axial skeleton and pain in at least 11 of 18 characteristic tender points

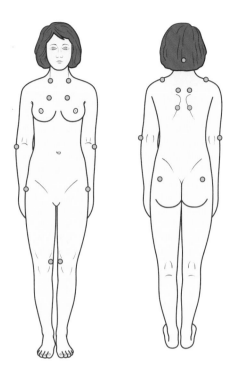

Figure 10.1 Classical tender points in fibromyalgia.

The terms 'fibrositis' and 'psychogenic rheumatism' have been used in the past to describe the same syndrome. Whether fibromyalgia is simply a continuum of pain and fatigue or a distinct disease entity remains controversial. Although an association with selective disturbance of alpha-delta sleep has been described, a relentless search for underlying pathology affecting muscles, the microcirculation, the nervous system and neuro-endocrine mechanisms has failed to reveal any convincing evidence of a clear aetiology. However, the concept of fibromyalgia as a syndrome of generalized heightened sensitivity to pain, possibly as a result at least in part to a deranged sleep pattern, is useful when considering approaches to management of the disorder.

Up to 90% of patients with fibromyalgia are women, mostly aged 30–60 years. The prevalence of the disorder varies geographically, with Caucasians most commonly affected. The variation between nations is also associated, in part, with differences in the recognition of the disorder as a distinct entity. In the USA, the prevalence is 2%, with an increasing prevalence with age.

Investigations aim primarily to exclude other conditions with a similar clinical picture (Table 10.2).

Management. Approaches to the management of fibromyalgia include education about the disorder, pain control, sleep modulation and physical conditioning.

Firm reassurance is a vital part of patient education, and an outline of the concepts surrounding the disorder should be given. Details of the management programme and appropriate expectations should be given. Involvement of the multidisciplinary team is necessary.

Exercise. In addition to patient education, exercise is recognized to be the mainstay of therapy for fibromyalgia. Aerobic exercise programmes have been shown to reduce tender point counts and physician global assessment

TABLE 10.2

Differential diagnoses and routine investigations in fibromyalgia

Differential diagnosis	Routine investigations
• Systemic lupus erythematosus	• Full blood count and white cell differential
• Rheumatoid arthritis	
• Sjögren's syndrome	• Erythrocyte sedimentation rate
• Polymyalgia rheumatica	• C-reactive protein
• Myositis	• Creatine kinase
• Hypothyroidism	• Renal, liver and bone biochemistry
• Neuropathies	
• Neoplasm, including lymphoproliferative disorders	• Thyroid function
	• Autoantibody screen and rheumatoid factor
• Others, e.g. borreliosis, Lyme disease	• Chest X-ray
	• B12 and folate*
*As indicated	• Nerve conduction studies*

scores. Counselling, encouragement and supervision are necessary for such programmes to succeed, as most patients initially feel that exercise will worsen their symptoms.

Pain control and sleep modulation can often be achieved by the use of tricyclic agents, such as dothiepin, usually in a single dose at bedtime. Patients must be warned that several weeks may elapse before an effect is noted. They should also be warned about potential side-effects, such as sedation in the morning, tremor, dizziness, dry mouth, weight gain and constipation. Note that morning sedation is common in the first few days but dose reduction may be necessary if it continues.

Other approaches to pain control, including the use of NSAIDs, offer no clinical benefit compared with that of simple analgesics. The use of opioids is generally discouraged. Acupuncture is usually unsuccessful in fibromyalgia and may exacerbate the problem (in contrast to its often beneficial effect in myofascial pain syndromes, see pages 86–7). Other non-pharmacological approaches to pain control, including hypnotherapy, biofeedback and cognitive–behavioural therapy have not shown significant benefit.

Prognosis. The few long-term, longitudinal studies performed in fibromyalgia indicate that the outlook is somewhat bleak, with many individuals reporting persisting pain and dysfunction. However, the majority report improvement since the time of diagnosis, with younger patients and those with lower initial pain scores having better outcomes. The incidence of long-term disability has been reported as 9–44%.

Regional myofascial pain syndromes

These are characterized by regional pain with associated trigger points (Figure 10.2). A trigger point is an area, usually muscular, of exquisite tenderness with an expanded receptive field of referred pain. The characteristics of trigger points are shown in Table 10.3. The relationship between trigger and tender points is unclear, and myofascial pain and fibromyalgia may simply represent two ends of a continuous spectrum.

Clinical features. Trigger points result in a decreased muscle stretch and pain on contraction. Contributing aetiological factors include traumatic and whiplash injuries, postural and repetitive strains, muscle tension

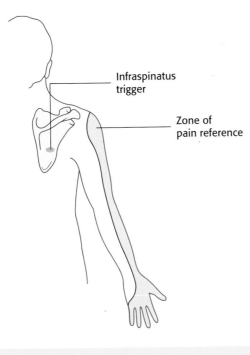

Infraspinatus
trigger

Zone of
pain reference

Figure 10.2 An example
of a trigger point.

TABLE 10.3

Characteristics of trigger points

- Localized, deep area of tenderness in a taut band of muscle
- Associated 'twitch response' of local muscle on palpation
- Palpation reproduces symptoms of pain locally and peripherally in a zone of reference

(producing habits), stress, sleep disturbance, deconditioning/disuse and physical illness.

Associated features include tension headaches, temporomandibular joint dysfunction, low back and neck pain, and gastrointestinal disturbance.

Management involves treatment of the trigger points (to break the pain cycle), muscle exercises and eradication of contributing factors. Trigger-point needling can be performed with a rapid, dry-needle approach, for example with acupuncture needles. Some practitioners favour injection of anaesthetic and/or steroid to the trigger point, although there is little evidence that this is more effective than dry needling alone. Stretching the taut band and spraying the area with cold spray prior to needling may also be beneficial.

Stretching, strengthening and conditioning exercises are used to condition the area and to re-educate posture.

CHAPTER 11
Future trends

Scientific understanding

The scientific understanding of soft tissue conditions is increasing slowly with the aid of new methodologies and application of new technologies. More research is necessary to characterize the heterogeneous cell populations now known to populate different soft tissues and to determine how these cells respond to injury. The interrelationships between ageing and other factors, such as mechanical stresses, hormones, growth factors and cytokines, and cell responses to injury need to be established.

Diagnosis

Advances in imaging technologies, such as MRI and ultrasound, have already led to significant improvements in the diagnosis of soft tissue pathology and these techniques are likely to become more sensitive, affordable and widely used in the objective assessment of individual conditions.

In the future, early changes in protein structure and composition may be monitored by non-invasive techniques, such as nuclear magnetic resonance spectroscopy. Biochemical analysis of tendon protein degradation products, released into the blood stream or synovial fluid, has allowed their investigation as potential markers for early tendon damage in horses, and a similar approach may be possible in human tendinopathies.

Future management and treatment

Increasingly, it is being recognized that evidence is lacking for benefit in many of the regimens commonly used in the management of soft tissue disorders. This is not necessarily because these approaches are ineffective, but research in the field is often poorly designed and results have added to confusion rather than contributing to improved patient care. Nevertheless, it is likely that such approaches will continue to be used until evidence for their effectiveness, or otherwise, is produced or superior treatments developed.

Based on the premise that much soft tissue pathology represents a failure to adequately repair tissue after injury, future treatment strategies may be targeted at improving the wound-healing response in these tissues.

There have been major advances in our understanding of wound healing in skin. If generally applicable to soft tissues, such as tendons and ligaments, these advances may result in new therapies. For example, growth factors, such as transforming growth factor-β, designed to promote regeneration of the tendon matrix structure and composition may be useful. An alternative strategy that may prove useful in the future involves gene therapy in tendon and ligament injuries.

When tissues are extensively damaged, such as in cruciate ligament rupture, currently there is no better option than to reconstruct the ligament, frequently using the central portion of the patient's own patellar tendon. The science of 'tissue engineering' is likely to have a major impact on the reconstruction of soft tissues. Methods are being developed to create whole tissues in culture that replicate the structure and composition of the original tissue. Cartilage, skin, ligaments and tendons have all been constructed from stem cells and supporting three-dimensional matrices, and in the future it may be possible to surgically transplant artificially grown ligaments and tendons into patients.

Key references

GENERAL

Sallis RE, Massimino F, eds. *ACSM's Essentials of Sports Medicine*. St Louis, Missouri: Mosby, 1996.

STRUCTURE AND PATHOLOGY

Jozsa L, Kannus P. *Human Tendons. Anatomy, Physiology and Pathology*. Champaign, Illinois: Human Kinetics, 1997.

Woo SL-Y, Buckwalter JA. *Injury and Repair of the Musculoskeletal Soft Tissues*. Illinois: American Academy of Orthopedic Surgeons, 1987.

PATHOPHYSIOLOGY AND EPIDEMIOLOGY

Clancy WG. Tendon trauma and overuse injuries. In: Leadbetter WB, Buckwater JA, Gordon SL, eds. *Sports Induced Inflammation*. Park Ridge, Illinois: American Academy of Orthopedic Surgeons, 1990.

Puddu G, Ippolitto E, Postacchini P. A classification of Achilles tendon disease. *Am J Sports Med* 1976;4:145–50.

IMAGING

Chhem RK, Cardinal E, eds. *Guidelines and Gammuts in Musculoskeletal Ultrasound*. New York: Wiley-Liss, 1999.

MANAGEMENT

Doherty M, Hazleman BL, Hutton CW et al. *Rheumatology Examination and Injection Techniques*. 2nd edn. London: WB Saunders, 1998.

el Hawary R, Stanish WD, Curwin SL. Rehabilitation of tendon injuries in sport. *Sports Med* 1997;24:347–58.

Fyfe I, Stanish WD. The use of eccentric training and stretching in the treatment and prevention of tendon injuries. *Clin Sports Med* 1992;11:601–24.

Jones JG, Hazleman RL. The prognosis and management of polymyalgia rheumatica. *Ann Rheum Dis* 1981; 40:1–5.

Stiell IG, McKnight RD, Greenberg GH et al. Implementation of the Ottawa Ankle Rules. *JAMA* 1994;271:827–32.

SHOULDER

Ciullo JV. *Shoulder Injuries in Sport. Evaluation, Treatment and Rehabilitation*. Champaign, Illinois: Human Kinetics, 1996.

Gam AN, Schydlowsky P, Rossel I et al. Treatment of 'frozen shoulder' with distension and glucocorticoid compared with glucocorticoid alone: a randomised controlled trial. *Scand J Rheumatol* 1998; 27:425–30.

Hazleman BL, Dieppe BL, eds. The shoulder joint. *Baillieres Clin Rheumatol* 1989;3:3.

Nevasier T. Arthrography of the shoulder. *Orthop Clin N Am* 1980;11:205–17.

Nevasier RJ, Nevasier TJ. The frozen shoulder. Diagnosis and management. *Clin Orthop* 1987;223:59–64.

Speed CA, Hazleman BL. Shoulder pain.
Clinical Evidence 2000;3:558–72.

FIBROMYALGIA AND REGIONAL MYOFASCIAL PAIN SYNDROMES

Masi AT, ed. Fibromyalgia and
myofascial pain syndromes. *Baillieres
Clin Rheumatol* 1994;8:4.

Travell JG, Simons DG. Myofascial pain
and dysfunction. In: *The Trigger Point
Manual.* Volumes 1 & 2. Baltimore:
Williams & Wilkins, 1992.

Wolfe F, Smythe HA, Yunus MB *et al.*
The American College of Rheumatology
1990 criteria for the classification of
fibromyalgia. Report of the Multicentre
Criteria Committee. *Arthritis Rheum*
1990;33:160–72.

Index